YES, YOU CAN!

A Guide to Self-Care
for Persons with
Spinal Cord Injury
THIRD EDITION

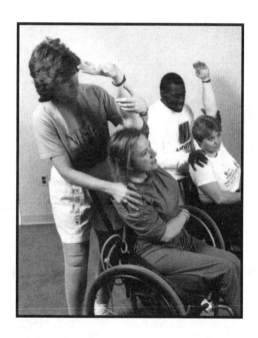

Edited By:

Margaret C. Hammond, MD
Stephen C. Burns, MD

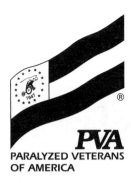

PVA
PARALYZED VETERANS
OF AMERICA

801 Eighteenth Street, NW
Washington, DC 20006-3517
(800) 424-8200
(800) 795-4327 TTY
www.pva.org

Library of Congress Cataloging-in-Publication Data
Paralyzed Veterans of America
Yes, You Can!
A Guide to Self-Care for Persons with Spinal Cord Injury
ISBN 0-929819-12-8   CIP 89-062035

A Word from the Paralyzed Veterans of America (PVA)

PVA would like to once again thank Dr. Margaret Hammond, as well as the other contributors to the 3rd edition of *Yes, You Can!* This edition has been expanded to include seven new chapters, including topics such as exercise, alternative medicine, pain, and substance abuse. We have also enhanced chapters to include additional resources and web sites. Another added feature is a list of organizations that can offer assistance in a variety of areas to people with spinal cord injury (SCI). Please note that the information on these web sites and resource organizations was accurate at the time of printing. We anticipate this manual to continue to be the best source of information in the SCI field.

This patient guide, *Yes, You Can! A Guide for Self-Care for Persons with Spinal Cord Injury*, was prepared by the Seattle Veterans Administration Medical Center (VAMC) Spinal Cord Injury Service in 1986. Written by experts at the center for the VAMC's spinal cord injury patient population, the guide was so successful that the center was unable to fulfill the many requests for copies that came from individuals outside the medical center. To make the benefits of this comprehensive manual available to a larger audience, the Seattle VAMC asked PVA to publish and distribute the manual.

Since PVA's inception more than 50 years ago, the organization's primary goal has been to maximize the quality of life for people with a spinal cord injury or disease through research, education, advocacy, and sports and recreation programs. *Yes, You Can!* was felt to be an outstanding project to further the educational needs of not only PVA members, but of all people with a spinal cord injury or disease.

The Board of Directors of PVA's Spinal Cord Injury Education and Training Foundation (ETF) agreed to fund the project as a specially targeted education and training activity. ETF is committed to patient/client education. This education gives the patient, family, and friends greater understanding of spinal cord injury and important life and health skills and, thus, helps the clients reach their maximum health potential.

The Seattle VAMC's manual, *Yes, You Can!*, has been reviewed and praised for its content, style, and presentation by individuals in the spinal cord injury field. Their suggestions for minor revisions have been incorporated, and the manual has been updated.

PVA believes this manual to be an important reference for the individual with a spinal cord injury on how to handle problems and where to turn for help. It is comprehensive and provides easy-to-read, practical knowledge on a large number of medical, psychological, social, and vocational issues.

Initially, the target audience for this manual was intended to be the newly injured SCI patient on the SCI unit; however, *Yes, You Can!* also has been popular with the out-of-hospital SCI population.

Paralyzed Veterans of America

Acknowledgments

A vote of thanks is owed to the following staff members of the Seattle VA Medical Center who were instrumental in the development of this education manual. As a team, this group of individuals contributed many hours of research and writing that produced the chapters contained herein.

Nicheole Amundsen, RN (Ch. 2, 3, 4, 6, 11 & 12)
Catherine Britell, MD (Ch. 1 & 10)
Diane Clowers, RN (Ch. 6)
Sue Davenport, MSW (Editorial assistance;
    Ch. 13, 15, 19 & 21)
Marguerite David, MSW (Ch. 13, 14, 15, 19 & 21)
Joel DeLisa, MD (Administrative Support;
    Ch. 1 & 10)
Sue Grogan, RN (Ch. 6, 7, 12 & 19)
Arne Hagen, Graphic Illustrator
Margaret Hammond, MD (Editor, Ch .3, 4, 11 & 12)
Jennifer Hunsaker-Young, RPT (Ch. 5)
Kaye Lawrence, RN, MSN (Ch. 2, 3 & 4)
Kathleen Linnell, MSN, Patient Education
    Coordinator
James Little, MD, PhD (Ch. 1 & 11)
Janet Loehr, RN, CRNP (Ch. 2, 4, 6, 7, 11 & 12)
Elizabeth Marsh, RPT (Ch. 5; ROM drawings)
Brenda Matteson (Editor; Project Coordinator;
    Ch. 9)
David McDonald, OTR (Editorial assistance;
    Ch. 5, 10, 12, 14, 18, 19, 20, 21)
Carolyn Neary, RD (Ch. 8)
Karen Ognan, RPT (Ch. 5 & 10)
Peggy O'Neil Freeman, VRS (Ch. 16)
Daniel Overton, CTRS (Ch. 17)
Sonya Perdita-Fulginiti, RN, MSN (Editor; Ch. 2, 6,
    7, 11 & 12)
Sue Pomeroy, OTR (Ch. 18 20)
Christina Scott, Graphic Designer
Kathy Stotts, PhD (Ch. 13 & 14)
Carole Sweetland, CTRS (Ch. 17)
Dale Tilly, Chief, Medical Media Production Service
Robert Umlauf, PhD (Editor; Ch. 13, 14, 15 & 19)

We would like to thank the many people who have contributed to this project with their positive feedback and constructive criticism.

Thanks also to the Seattle VA facility and to Dana Alskog and Tim Heritage, the people who volunteered for the photographs.

Special thanks to the Paralyzed Veterans of America, Rebecca Sadin, and Catherine Britell, MD, for their roles in the final publication of this book.

Acknowledgments for the Second Edition

Thank you to Janet Loehr, ARNP; Richard Buhrer, CRRN; Jennifer Hunsaker-Young, PT; Laura Sapp, COTA/L; and Marguerite David, MSW, for their contributions to this edition. As always, thanks to the team members of the Seattle VAMC Spinal Cord Injury Service for their comprehensive and compassionate care to our patients

Margaret C. Hammond, MD, Editor

Acknowledgments for the Third Edition

Many of the chapters in this third edition are an update of content included in the first two editions; some chapters are new. A heartfelt thank you is extended to the following members of the VA Puget Sound Health Care System spinal cord injury team for their contributions to this edition:

Kendra Betz, MS, PT (Ch. 24)
Richard Buhrer, MN, RN, CRRN (Ch. 27)
Stephen P. Burns, MD (Ch. 3)
Diane E. Clowers, RN (Ch. 6 & 14)
Thomas M. Collins, MPT (Ch. 5)
Pat Custer, RN, ADN, CRRN (Ch. 4)
Marguerite J. David, MSW, CSW (Ch. 13, 15,
    19 & 21)
Elaine Detwiler, RN, BSN, CRRN (Ch. 4)
Stephen G. Fitzgerald, PhD (Ch. 14 &23)
L. Paige Fritz, MS, RD (Ch. 8)
Randee Frost, BSOT (Ch. 26)
Jennifer Hastings, MSPT (Ch. 5)
Laura Heard, CRRN, MS (Ch. 2)
Jennifer James, MD (Ch. 9 & 25)
James W. Little, MD, PhD (Ch. 1 & 22)
Patty J. Lyman, PA-C, BS (Ch. 11)
Anthony J. Mariano, PhD (Ch. 23)
Peggy O'Neil Freeman, MEd (Ch. 16)
Wannapha Petchkrua, MD (Ch. 22)
Tammy Pidde, CRRN, BSN (Ch. 2 &7)
Leilani Redosendo, RN, BSN, CRRN (Ch. 4)
Elaine M. Rogers Fanucchi, MSPT (Ch. 10 & 26)
Cathy Rundell, CRRN, BSN (Ch. 2)
Darci L. Sgrignoli, MS, OTR/L (Ch. 20)
Mary Anne Smith, CRRN, BSN (Ch. 2)
Steven A. Stiens, MD, MS (Ch. 7)
Sandy Symons, AS (Ch. 26)
David Tostenrude, MPA, CTRS (Ch. 17)
Teresa Valois, BS-OT, OTR/L CDRS (Ch. 18)
Claire C. Yang, MD (Ch. 6 & 14)

Thanks to Steven Stiens, MD, for his review as a professional and consumer. Additional thanks to Dianne D'Alessandro for her skillful ability in leading this project to fruition.

Special thanks to the Paralyzed Veterans of America staff, Andrea Censky Dietrich, Joan Napier, James Angelo, Chris Campbell, and Patricia Scully, for designing, editing, and coordinating publication of this book.

Margaret C. Hammond, MD, Editor, 3rd Edition
Stephen C. Burns, MD, Co-Editor, 3rd Edition

Contents

Here's to Your Independence!

The goal of rehabilitation is to help you design a lifestyle that will allow you to function as independently as possible within the realm of your ability.

This manual has been put together to help you. It covers many things you learn while you are in the hospital.

When you get home, the manual will serve as a resource for what you have learned. The information is there to answer any questions that may arise about caring for yourself. This manual does not replace your SCI clinic or physician. If you really get in a jam, call your nearest SCI center.

Spinal Cord Anatomy & Physiology

Even though the brain controls the majority of the activities of your body, it only extends down as far as the top of your neck. Beyond that, the *spinal cord* takes over and acts like telephone wires for messages coming and going between the brain and all the other parts of your body. Your face has a direct connection to the brainstem, so it is independent of your spinal cord.

The spinal cord looks like a long, rope-like cord about the width of your little finger. It runs from the base of your brain down to the lower part of your back and it is fairly fragile. Damage to your spinal cord can affect your ability to move or feel. It can also affect the workings of some internal organs. If you are injured at a given level of your spinal cord, parts of your body will be affected at and below that level.

To avoid damage, the spinal cord is protected by bone—specifically, by your *back bones* or spine. The back bones are 29 small bones stacked one on top of the other. These bones are called *vertebrae (VERT-i-bray).*

FIGURE 1.1. The Spinal Column

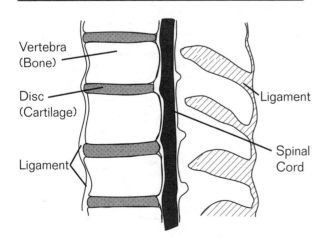

Vertebra (Bone)

Disc (Cartilage)

Ligament

Ligament

Spinal Cord

Because of all the jarring and bending your back must do, each *vertebra (VERT-i-brah)* is cushioned from the next by *disks*. Disks are made of spongy material that act like shock absorbers. Ligaments hold the vertebrae together and allow your neck and back to twist and bend.

Each vertebra has a hole in it, so when vertebrae are stacked together, they provide a hard, bony tunnel through which the spinal cord passes. This is called the spinal column. In this way, the spinal cord is protected from damage. *(See figure 1.1.)*

There are four sections of your spine. The top is the *cervical (SURR-vick-ull)* section, which makes up your neck. The next down is the *thoracic (thor-ASS-ick)* section, which runs to your waist level. The *lumbar (LUMM-bar)* level is next and is your lower back. And last is the *sacral (SAY-crull)* part, which is your tailbone. *(See figure 1.2.)*

There are eight pairs of nerves and seven vertebrae in the cervical section of your spine. In this case, the nerves numbered C1 through C7 are above the corresponding numbered vertebrae. C8 then slips through between the C7 and T1 bones. For the thoracic and lumbar sections, each of the numbered nerves lies below the corresponding numbered vertebra. There are 12 thoracic vertebrae and 5 lumbar vertebrae.

At the lower end of your spinal cord (below the second lumbar vertebra), the nerves travel long distances before they exit the spine. This is because the spinal cord itself ends much higher than where your tailbone marks the lower end of your spine.

This makes the lower lumbar and sacral nerves look like a horse's tail inside the spinal column. It is known as the *cauda equina (CODD-ah eh-QUINE-ah)*, which means "horse's tail" in Latin.

Your sacral section is really only one piece of bone with five nerve pairs coming out through holes in it.

WHAT THE SPINAL CORD DOES

The spinal cord is the communicating link between the *spinal nerves* and the brain. The nerves that lie only within the spinal cord itself are called *upper motor neurons (UMNs)*. These run only between the brain and the spinal nerves. The spinal nerves branch out from the spinal cord into the tissues of your body. Spinal nerves are also called *lower motor neurons (LMNs)*. *(See figure 1.3.)*

In movement, the brain sends messages through the spinal cord (UMNs) to the spinal nerves (LMNs). The LMNs then carry these messages to the muscles to coordinate complicated movements such as walking. In this way, the brain can influence movement.

In sensation, information is collected by nerves in your body and sent up the spinal cord to the brain. This allows conscious awareness of feelings such as heat or cold.

You may wonder how the spinal cord keeps these messages from getting confused, with all the running back and forth between

FIGURE 1.2. The Spinal Cord

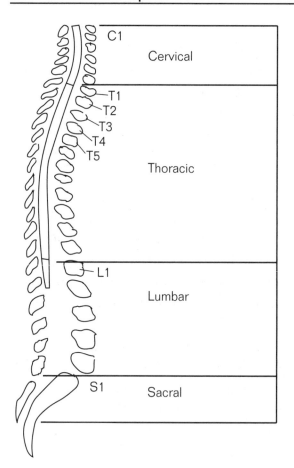

FIGURE 1.3. Spinal Nerves

LMNs connect the spinal cord (UMNs) with muscles, blood vessels, glands, organs, etc.

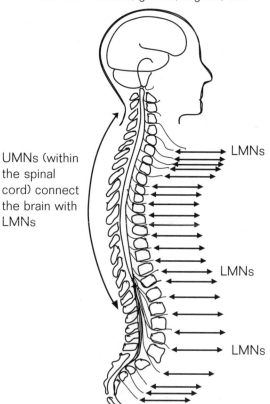

UMNs (within the spinal cord) connect the brain with LMNs

LMNs

LMNs

LMNs

brain and body. The motor nerves and the sensory nerves carry messages in different nerve fibers.

Within the cord itself, the nerve fibers are combined into *spinal tracts*. Each tract carries messages one way, either up for sensation or down for voluntary movement. They are similar to the lanes on a freeway. *(See figure 1.4.)*

What Is a Spinal Nerve and What Does It Do?

Each spinal nerve has two main parts. One part carries information related to movement from the spinal cord to the muscles. It is called the *motor* portion of the nerve. Each motor portion of a spinal nerve connects to a specific muscle group. Each level of the spinal cord causes movement in a corresponding group of muscles.

The other part of the spinal nerve carries messages of feeling, such as heat and cold, from the body to the spinal cord. It is called the sensory portion of the nerve.

Different types of sensation or feeling are carried up the spinal cord to the brain. These include pain, touch, heat, cold, vibration, pressure, and knowing where a body part is located in space without looking at it.

Each sensory portion of the spinal nerve collects information about feelings from a given area of skin. Each area is called a *dermatome (DER-muh-tome)* and matches a specific spinal cord level. *(See figure 1.5.)*

FIGURE 1.5. Map of Dermatomes

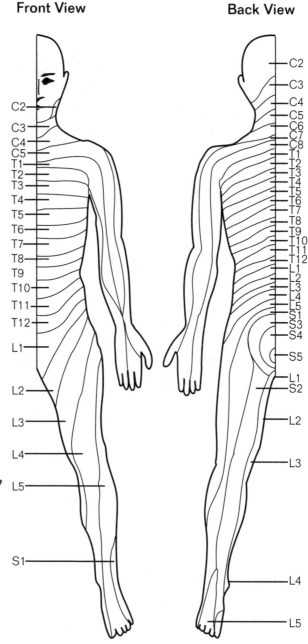

FIGURE 1.4. Spinal Tracts for Nerves

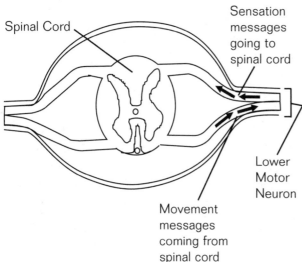

FIGURE 1.6. Your Own Dermatome Map

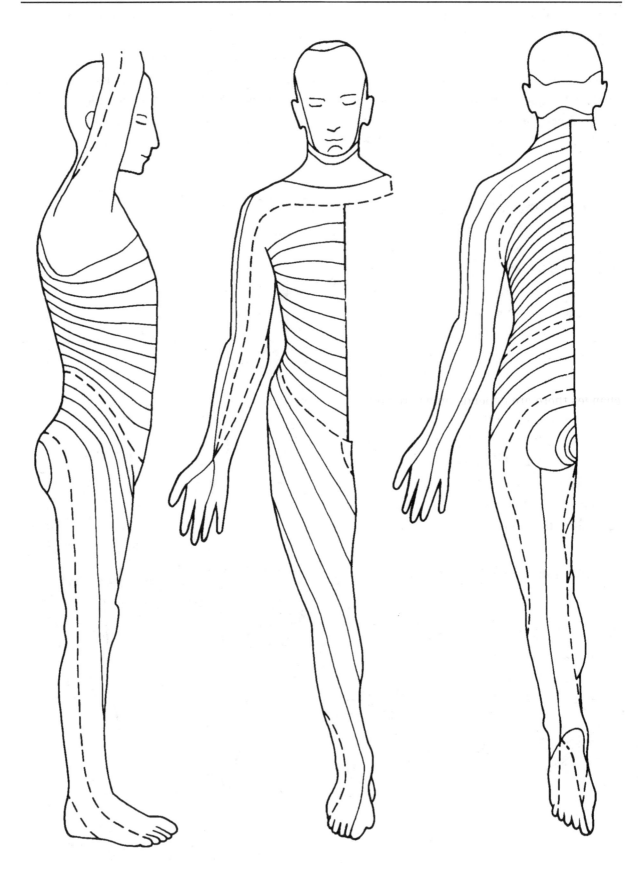

You might want to make your own map of dermatome sensation using the blank map (*figure 1.6*). Color in the sections where you have feeling. See if the map can tell you your level of injury.

SPINAL CORD INJURY (SCI)

Excessive movement of vertebrae often causes a spinal cord injury. When bones in your back and neck are broken or when ligaments are torn, the spinal cord can get squeezed between two vertebrae. Sometimes stab wounds or gunshot wounds can damage the cord without breaking bones.

Damage to your spinal cord can cause changes in your movement, feeling, bladder control, or other bodily functions. How many changes there are depends on where your spinal cord was injured and how severely the spinal cord was injured. The main problem is that the connection between your brain and the parts of your body below the injury is impaired.

A numbering system is used to name levels of injury. It is the same as the system used to name bone and nerve levels in your back. A spinal cord injury is named for the lowest level of the spinal cord that still functions the way it did before your injury. It is important to your rehabilitation that you know your level of injury and how it affects your body.

Complete and Incomplete SCI

When there is no voluntary movement (spasms don't count—they are involuntary) or feeling below your spinal cord injury level, you have a *complete injury*.

If you do have some feeling or voluntary movement below your injury, you have an *incomplete injury*. This happens when there

is only partial damage to your spinal cord; that is, some nerve fibers are preserved across your spinal cord injury site.

Upper Motor Neuron (UMN) and Lower Motor Neuron (LMN) Injuries

Earlier in this chapter, we discussed the difference between upper motor neurons (UMNs) and lower motor neurons (LMNs). This section will tell you why it is important that you know this.

Most spinal injuries damage both UMNs and LMNs. A complete injury cuts or squeezes all the UMNs running down the spinal cord. This disrupts the connection between the brain and the parts of the body below the injury. LMNs below your spinal cord injury are not damaged. Because LMNs carry reflex actions, the reflexes below the level of injury are still in working order. This is a *UMN injury. (See figure 1.7.)*

The reflex action that the LMNs carry out below the level of injury may still work, but there is one problem. In reflexes, the brain keeps control on how much your nerves react. In a UMN injury, control by the brain no longer exists because messages from the brain can't get through the point of injury. The LMNs act by themselves, causing reflexes without limit. One example is spasticity (spa-STI-si-ti). Spasticity is the uncontrolled movement of your arms or legs. See more about spasticity in the chapter on "Nerves, Muscles & Bones."

LMN injuries are a different story. This kind of injury is found for the most part at the lower tip of the spinal cord, or the cauda equina. Damage to the cauda equina impairs reflex actions. This is because the cauda equina is made up entirely of LMNs. Other UMNs and LMNs above the injury are still in good shape. *(See figure 1.8.)*

FIGURE 1.7. Upper Motor Neuron Injury

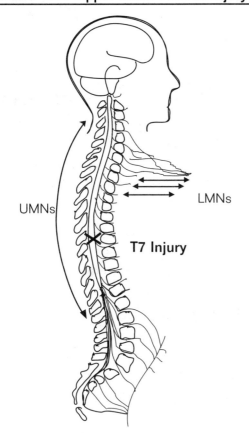

UMNs

LMNs

T7 Injury

FIGURE 1.8. Lower Motor Neuron Injury

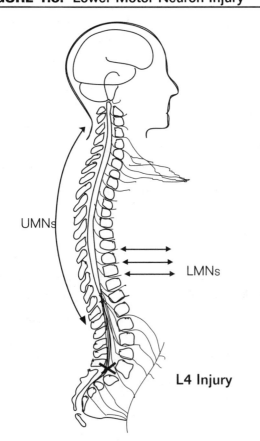

UMNs

LMNs

L4 Injury

Spasticity is not found in LMN injuries as it is in UMN injuries, because muscles governed by these LMNs tend to shrink or *atrophy (AT-row-fee)*. This is because these muscles no longer have any nerve contact to stimulate them.

Stated simply, a *UMN injury* is one where the UMN pathway is broken and the LMNs below the injury are intact and spasticity is noted. An *LMN injury*, usually at the cauda equina, abolishes nerve contact with muscles controlled below the injury and no spasticity develops. It is important for you to know which type of injury you have, because how your spinal cord injury is managed will differ depending on that fact.

RECOVERY

Immediately after a spinal cord injury, the spinal cord stops doing its job for a period of time called "spinal shock." All the reflexes below the level of injury are absent during this period of several weeks or months. The return of reflexes below the level of injury marks the end of spinal shock. At this time, your doctor can determine if you have a complete or an incomplete injury.

If you have an incomplete injury, some feelings and movement may come back. *Will this happen to you?* No one can say. If you do regain some feeling and movement, it will likely start in the first few weeks after your injury.

Rehabilitation begins immediately. You will be instructed in strengthening exercises, new styles of movement, and the use of special equipment to work with what you have. If you do get additional recovery of feeling or movement, your rehabilitation team will develop new goals with you.

Skin covers and protects your entire body. It is made up of two layers of tissue: the *epidermis (epp-a-DURR-miss)* and the *dermis (DURR-miss).*

The *epidermis*, or surface layer, consists of an outer part of dead cells and an inner part of living cells. The outer part of the epidermis acts as a buffer between the underlying body tissues and the environment. Dead cells are constantly shed and replaced with newer ones from the inner part of the epidermis.

The *dermis*, or under layer of the skin, consists of thick fibrous tissue that gives strength and elasticity to the skin. It contains hair follicles (roots), sweat glands, *sebaceous (sub-AY-shuss)* or oil glands, blood vessels, and nerve endings. *(See figure 2.1.)*

FIGURE 2.1. Skin

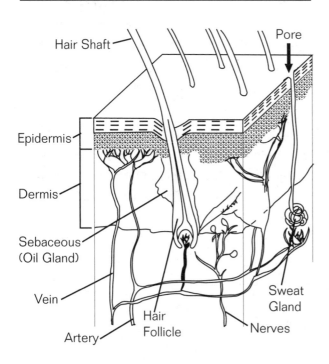

WHAT SKIN DOES

The four functions of your skin are:

- Protection
- Sensation
- Fluid regulation
- Temperature regulation

Your skin does this for all of the body structures and tissues beneath it. This includes layers of fat, muscles, and bones.

- Your skin serves as a *shield* against most forms of chemical and physical agents, such as bacteria, dirt, foreign objects (such as pebbles), and ultraviolet rays from the sun.

- The skin also has a *sensory* function. The sensations of touch, pain, and temperature travel from nerve endings in your skin through the spinal cord to your brain.

- A major function of the skin is *regulation of your body fluids and temperature.* Sweat glands are always producing water and salts, changing the fluid content of your body. When liquid from your sweat glands evaporates, it helps maintain a stable body temperature.

Table 2.A shows how these functions of the skin are affected by a spinal cord injury and what you need to do to prevent problems.

WHY YOU SHOULD WORRY ABOUT PRESSURE

Adequate circulation of your blood is needed to keep the cells of your skin and body tissues alive. When your circulation is cut off for a prolonged time, cells die and sores develop.

TABLE 2.A. How Skin Is Affected by SCI and How to Prevent These Problems

FUNCTIONS	CHANGE	YOU NEED TO
Protection	No change.	Avoid breaks in your skin.
Sensation	Decrease in or no feeling of touch, pain, and temperature below the level of your SCI.	Substitute specific protective habits to prevent injury to skin and underlying tissues.
Temperature Regulation	Less sweat to evaporate and cool you below the level of your SCI.	Control temperature of your environment (stay out of sun, maybe use air conditioning). When in the sun, drink plenty of fluids.
	May have excessive sweating above the level of your SCI.	Bathe more frequently. Possibly take medication.
Fluid Regulation	No voluntary muscle action below the level of your SCI can produce swelling of the tissues due to pooling of fluids (edema).	Elevate swollen parts to reduce edema. Wear compressive stockings.

These sores are called *pressure sores* (decubitus or "decubs").

Pressure can come from outside of your body, such as from the seat of your wheelchair or from the mattress on your bed. The pressure of your weight pushes your bones onto blood vessels, especially in areas where bones normally stick out somewhat. The blood vessels become trapped between the outside surface and your bones and get closed off. *(See figure 2.2.)* Blood, which carries oxygen and nutrients, cannot get past that point. Unless the pressure is relieved, the cells that are fed by those blood vessels will die, and a sore will form. Be aware that this kind of problem can develop in as short a time as 30 minutes.

Regular *pressure releases* when you are up in your wheelchair or position changes when you are lying down will allow the blood vessels to open again and prevent skin breakdown. Fortunately, pressure causes changes in your skin that provide *early warning signs* that the cells are not getting adequate circula-

tion. These early warning signs of damage are *redness and firmness*.

Shearing

Shearing occurs when two layers of tissue right next to each other are pulled in opposite directions. This can also lead to skin tears and breakdown. The blood vessels in the layers of the skin are closed off by the pulling. *(See figure 2.3.)*

Shearing can happen if you slip down in your wheelchair. It also can happen when you sit in bed. If the head of your bed is elevated, you may slide down, which then can lead to shearing at the sacrum.

Shearing plus direct pressure from the weight of your body increases your risk of getting pressure sores.

Friction on Your Skin

Friction produced from constant rubbing or pulling of your skin across surfaces can cause blisters. It should be avoided. Friction

FIGURE 2.2. Pressure on Skin

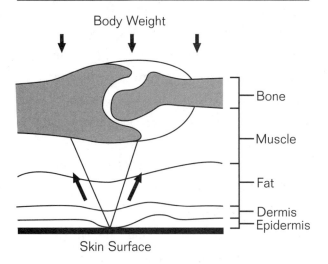

Skin Surface

FIGURE 2.3. Shearing

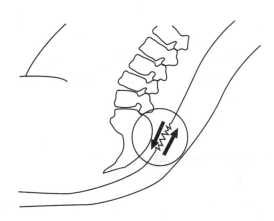

occurs when you drag any body part across a bed, toilet, or other surface during a transfer. Friction can also be caused by spasms. Your heels are a common site for this problem.

Dealing with Pressure Sores

Successful treatment of pressure sores requires removing the cause.

- Remove all pressure.
- Keep off the pressure sore.
- Keep the area around your sore clean and dry.
- May require bedrest with no sitting.

There are different ways to manage pressure sores after they have developed. Some may even require surgical repair. You may need a referral to a visiting nurse agency to help you heal your wound. All ways of treating pressure sores take a long time to work and require keeping pressure off the area. If you develop a pressure sore, talk with your nurse or doctor about it. Please see the chapter "Pressure Sores" for further information.

SKIN CARE

Nutrition for the Skin

Vitamins A, C, E, and B6 or *niacin (NIGH-ah-sinn)* are some key vitamins that are necessary for proper development and maintenance of healthy skin. These vitamins cannot function alone. They require adequate protein, calories, and other vitamins and minerals to carry out their function. These nutrients can be obtained by eating a well-balanced diet and a variety of foods. Some tips on how to eat a well-balanced diet can be found in the chapter on "Nutrition."

Weight Control

Weight control is another area of concern for skin care. Being at an appropriate weight for your height may help lower your risk for skin breakdowns. To get an idea of what an appropriate weight for your height is or if you are underweight or overweight, see the chapter on "Nutrition" for tips on how to achieve your ideal weight.

Basic Hygiene

We all need *regular hygiene (HIGH-jean)*. Dirt and grime, which normally contain different kinds of germs, settle on the surface of your skin. The total area of skin surface is approximately one square yard, which is a lot of breeding ground for tiny germs. Any cuts or scrapes of the skin will give these germs easy entry inside your body. Therefore, regular cleansing with soap and water by taking showers, tub baths, bed baths, or sponge baths is needed.

Daily bathing is encouraged during your younger and middle years. However, as you age, your skin becomes drier so daily whole body cleaning is not recommended. Skin should still be washed any time it is soiled. Areas such as armpits and groin still need daily cleaning.

Hygiene Tips Specific to SCI

Sitting in a wheelchair all day long with frequent weight shifts doesn't give air much of a chance to freely circulate in the groin area. Also, having your legs close together most of the day gives those normal body germs what they like most—a nice warm, dark, moist place to reproduce. And, if you're wearing some sort of plastic or rubber urine collecting device, such as condom catheter, foley catheter, waterproof padding, or leg bag, the chance of making that breeding ground more enticing to germs increases.

Hygiene Tips

1. Wash your groin area again before going to bed for the night.

2. Air out your groin area at least once a day by getting into the frog position.

3. Always thoroughly dry your groin area and in between your toes after bathing.

4. If you use powder, lightly dust some on your groin area. Be careful not to put on a lot. Too much powder can cake and cause lumps that could lead to irritation, rashes,

and splits in your skin. Or you may also try using a stick antiperspirant along your groin creases to control the moisture.

5. Clean your urine collecting equipment every day. See the chapter on "Bladder Management" for more information.

6. Apply lotion daily to dry skin areas, except between your toes unless your doctor instructs you to do so. Dry skin can crack open.

7. When doing nail care:
   • Clean finger and toe nails daily.
   • Keep your nails short for safety.
   • Cut your toe nails straight across to prevent ingrown nails.
   • Cut your nails after soaking them for 15-20 minutes or after taking a bath. This makes them easier to cut.
   • Thick nails may need to be cut by a podiatrist or clinic nurse.

DAILY SKIN CARE SPECIFIC TO SCI

You need to give your skin special attention every day because of the decrease in circulation, lack of feeling, and lack of movement in your body below the level of your injury. Pressure sores can develop quickly. The need to recognize, treat, and, most of all, *prevent* them is very important. Examining your skin for possible problems is essential.

Tips for Skin Inspection

1. Check your skin twice a day. Before you get out of bed, inspect those areas that have had pressure when you were lying down. After you get into bed, inspect those areas that have had pressure when you were sitting. (*See figure 2.4.*)

FIGURE 2.4. Skin Inspection Points

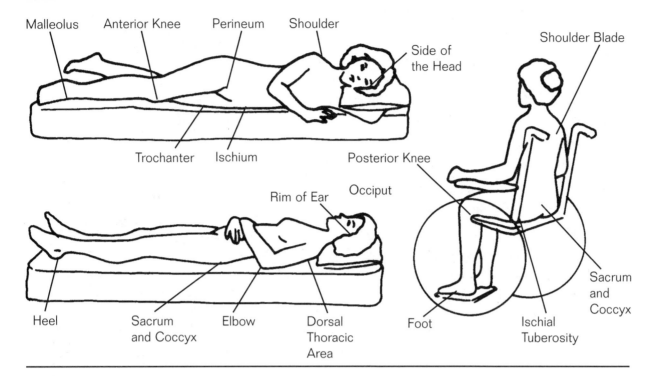

2. Check *all* your bony places (ankles, elbows, heels, hips, tailbone) below the level of your injury. Use a mirror to see those bony areas behind you, like your sitting bones.

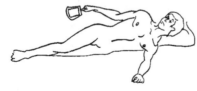

3. If you cannot use a mirror or check your skin yourself, get someone (like your attendant) to check those areas for you.

4. Look for reddened areas, cuts, scrapes, blisters, and bruises. Anything that seems different needs to be carefully checked out.

5. If you find a reddened area, check the "Troubleshooting" section of this chapter for what to do next.

6. Feel over the bony areas for changes like lumps or spots that are firmer than the rest of the skin around it.

Areas to Check

It is important to check the fit of your clothes, shoes, and equipment to be certain they are not too tight. Especially check the following items:

1. Thick seams, especially on blue jeans.

2. Binding in the groin area with pressure on your scrotum.

3. Tight shoes, especially if you have swollen feet.

4. Socks with elastic tops that bind around your lower leg.

5. Straps holding your urine drainage system that are too tight.

6. Condoms that have been applied too tightly.

Avoid These Problems

1. Wash clothing that you have never worn before wearing and check your skin after one or two hours for redness or chafing.

2. Buy jeans that are designed with low-profile seams (not bulky). Consider removing back pockets or buying jeans without them.

3. Buy jeans and slacks in a size larger than your usual size to prevent constriction.

4. If you are male, adjust your scrotum after you get dressed and transfer to your chair. Be certain that you are not sitting directly on your scrotum.

5. Unless compression socks have been prescribed, wear socks that are neither too tight nor too loose.

6. Check the fit of shoes carefully and watch your feet for signs of edema (swelling). After you have worn your shoes for 6 months or more, re-check the interior cushioning for signs of the padding wearing down.

7. Loosen or change the position of your urine drainage system.

POSITIONING/TURNING

Changing your body posture takes pressure off of your bony prominences. Listed below are some helpful tips for positioning/turning.

In Bed

1. *Change your position according to your skin tolerance level.* Use the routine of side to side to back for turns. Sleep on your stomach (prone), if possible. Note positioning of body parts and the use of pillows in the diagrams shown. *(See figure 2.5.)*

   • When lying on your back in bed, avoid pressure on your heels by "suspending" your feet over the edge of a pillow. Some people wear special foot splints to protect the skin over the ankles or heels.

FIGURE 2.5. Positioning/Turning in Bed

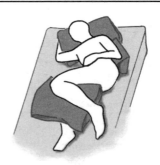

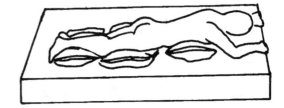

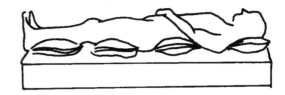

   • Side-lying pressure on the fleshy part of your buttock will protect the skin over your hip bone (trochanter).

   • Sitting in bed for prolonged periods is hazardous to the skin over your tail bone (sacrum, coccyx). So raise the head of the bed for short functional activities only.

2. *Use an alarm clock at first* to wake you for your turns. After a while, turning in bed may become automatic for you.

3. *Get someone else to turn you* (like your attendant) if you cannot do it for yourself.

4. You may need a specialized mattress. Please discuss with your doctor or nurse.

In a Wheelchair

1. *Do pressure releases every 15 minutes* to take the pressure off your tailbone and sitting bones. Ask your physical therapist

for a set of diagrams of pressure-release methods.

Your options are listed below. Work with your therapist to find which is best for you.

• Push up out of the seat of your wheelchair with your hands slightly forward and hold for 30-60 seconds.

• Lean side to side staying in a side-leaning position for 30-60 seconds per tilt.

• Bend your chest forward onto your knees and hold this position for 30-60 seconds

• Tilt your wheelchair back or use your recliner if you have one. Remain reclined for 1-2 minutes Some people have developed skin problems when they remained in a reclined position for long periods of time (greater than 30 minutes).

• Shift your position as much as possible. Be a wiggle worm. It doesn't come automatically, but constant moving allows the blood to continue flowing.

2. *Check your posture* by looking at yourself in a full length mirror after you are up in your wheelchair. Make sure that your ankles, the sides of your knees, and your hip bones are not leaning up against parts of your wheelchair. Your body has a natural balance and symmetry to it. Your knees and feet should appear to be "even." Spasticity and muscle strength imbalances can disrupt this balance and cause a change in your posture. Tight muscles in your trunk and legs can do the same. *Things to look out for include:*

• A curving or twisting of your back (spine).

• Tightness of your legs or your trunk that prevents your body from keeping its normal balance.

• One knee looking like it is "higher" than the other.

• Any appearance of "slumping" or leaning to one side of the wheelchair or the other.

3. *Make sure your foot pedals are adjusted for your height.*

4. Sit up as straight as possible in your wheelchair.

5. *Always use a WELL-MAINTAINED cushion.*

6. Be aware that any change in your positioning to ease pressure from one area will affect the pressure put on other areas.

PREVENTING INJURY

Before your spinal cord injury, your sensation warned you to move away from harm. Of course, accidents were always a possibility and will continue to be so.

After your spinal cord injury, you have lost some or all of the ability to feel and/or move below your level of injury. This puts you at risk for injury to your skin.

Tips for Preventing Injury:

1. Always be aware of how close your paralyzed body parts are to possible hazards around you. *Example:* Are they too close to a heater, fireplace, campfire, or exposed hot water pipes? After transferring to an overstuffed chair, are your feet squarely on the floor?

2. When transferring or moving around, be careful not to bump into things. Use your eyes to check out distances and obstacles. *Remember* that when you turn around in your wheelchair your feet stick out farther than the rest of you, so wear shoes to protect your toes.

3. Don't do fancy or new maneuvers in your wheelchair until you have been trained.

4. Spasms can lead to skin trauma. For example, a spasm during a tilt back can result in your ankle hitting a calf rest pad and causing injury.

5. Do not sleep in your wheelchair, because you cannot do a pressure release if you are asleep.

POTENTIAL HAZARDS TO SKIN

Alcohol Abuse

Many people drink alcohol. Alcohol and other drug use may impair your judgment, which may lead to accidents or other activities that can injure you and your skin. When people are intoxicated, they forget to do pressure releases, so they are at risk for pressure sores.

Solutions

1. To maintain clear thinking and good judgment, limit your alcohol intake. For example drink alcohol only during meals and limit yourself to one or two drinks a day (1 drink = 12 oz. of beer, 6 oz. of wine, 1 oz. hard liquor.) Please see the chapter on "Nutrition."

2. Do not drive a vehicle after drinking alcohol. Do not ride as a passenger in a vehicle driven by someone else who has been drinking alcohol.

3. If alcohol or drug use is difficult to control, consult your health-care provider, a local mental health center, or a community alcohol treatment program.

Anemia

Anemia (ah-NEEM-ee-ah) is the medical term to describe a decreased number of red blood cells (RBCs). Almost all (97%) of the oxygen that gets to your tissues is carried there by your RBCs. If your RBCs are low, you are *anemic (ah-NEEM-ick)*. If you do not have enough RBCs to carry oxygen to your cells, your skin is more prone to break down and, if it does break down, will be difficult to heal.

Solutions

There are many causes of anemia. One common cause of anemia is the lack of iron in your diet. You might try eating more red meats and green leafy vegetables or taking a vitamin with an iron supplement. You may benefit from consulting with a dietitian.

Cold Injuries

Your SCI puts you at risk for injury from things that are too cold because of the loss of skin sensation.

Solutions

1. Beware of frozen foods on your lap. Use a pad underneath frozen items.

2. If using ice over an area for swelling, wrap the ice in a towel. Do not ice longer than 10 minutes.

3. Prevent frostbite by wearing warm socks and sturdy shoes when outside. Cover your head, ears, and hands when you go out. If your ears are becoming numb and tingling, your feet probably are too, so come inside!

Hot Injuries

Your SCI puts you at risk for injury from things that are too hot because of the loss of skin sensation.

Solutions

1. Check the water temperature by putting a hand or other body part with feeling into the water and holding it there for five seconds. If you feel comfortable, the water temperature is safe. If you don't have good

sensation in your hand, have someone else check the water temperature or use a thermometer. Water temperature should typically range between 100° and 104° F for bathing.

2. Be sure your hot water heater is not set higher than 120° F. Scalding burns occur very rapidly at temperatures greater than 120° F.

3. Do not use a heating pad.

4. Beware of feet being too near the heater of a car.

5. Do not use electric blankets.

6. Do not move too close to fireplaces, radiators, hot water pipes (especially under sink), or campfires.

7. Do not carry hot fluids or foods in your lap without a tray. If you carry hot foods, use a sturdy board that covers the entire surface of the dish or pan to prevent burns from the hot container touching your leg.

8. Use cup holders on your wheelchair.

9. Do not fill cups too full.

10. Keep pan handles over the stove surfaces to prevent bumping them.

11. Do not wear loose-fitting long-sleeved shirts or reach across hot stove burners.

If you should burn yourself, initiate first aid treatment immediately. Apply cool water. Do not use ice or other frozen things on a burn.

If you spill hot food or fluids on yourself, you may not be able to detect all the places it came in contact with as it spilled. Pay close attention to your groin and buttocks areas.

Depression

For our definition, depression is not the feeling we all get from time to time of being down, gloomy, teary, or just fed up. A depressed person is someone who does not eat much, has no appetite, cannot sleep at night, or sleeps all the time. Depressed people also generally are very inactive and may neglect their self-care.

Depression itself does not cause problems to the skin, but the side effects of poor eating, sleeping, and not being active increase the likelihood of developing pressure sores from lack of movement.

Solutions

If you are just having a down day or two, don't worry. It is normal and will probably pass. If it continues for longer than that, call your health-care provider and ask to talk to the psychologist or your nurse or doctor. Get help if your mood does not improve.

Stress

It is common for many people to become tense, nervous, or worried by the demands of their daily activities. Muscle tension, increased blood pressure, irritability, and fatigue are common symptoms of stress.

With constantly raised blood pressure and muscle tension, your body uses more energy, tires easily, and uses up the vitamins, minerals, and nutrients needed for healthy skin.

Solutions

1. Read the chapter on "Psychosocial Adjustment." It has a section that describes relaxation, time management, and stress reduction.

2. Try to reduce your general stress level by taking time to relax every day.

Diabetes

Insulin is needed to get sugar into the cells for cell nutrition. When insulin is insufficient, sugar cannot get into the cells, and it builds up in the blood. That is why *glucose*

(GLUE-kose), or blood sugar, is elevated in people who have diabetes.

Diabetes damages blood vessels and nerves. It can cause decreases in sensation in the hands and feet, which can lead to wounds. When a person has diabetes, wounds are more likely to become infected, and they heal much slower.

Solutions

1. Control your blood sugar through diet, exercise, and use of medication if prescribed. Check your blood sugars as often as your health-care provider recommends.

2. Inspect your skin closely for reddened areas, blisters, or sores. Pay particular attention to your feet and legs.

3. Diabetic feet and toes are especially vulnerable to sores. Keep them clean and dry and your toenails trimmed. A tiny cut can lead to serious problems, so be careful to prevent injury.

4. If you get a reddened area or sore, cover it to protect it from further injury. If the sore does not heal in one week after following the troubleshooting suggestions at the end of this chapter, call your health-care provider.

Edema

Edema (eh-DEEM-ah) is a condition in which fluid collects in and around tissues. It is seen as swelling, usually of the feet and ankles and sometimes in the hands if you are a quadriplegic.

If tissues swell too much, it is hard to get adequate oxygen and nutrients to the cells. That increases the likelihood of skin breakdown. If you do get a sore, it takes longer to heal because of the decreased supply of oxygen and nutrients.

Solutions

1. Elevate your hands, legs, and feet frequently if these parts are affected.

2. Wear your compression stockings or gloves if they are prescribed.

3. Buy shoes one size larger to allow for swelling. Be aware of the amount of room from top to bottom in your shoe, not just the additional length, if you are prone to edema.

4. Make sure your braces, splints, clothing, and urinary devices are not too tight, causing constriction.

If the edema continues and you want to know more, see the edema section in the chapter on "Circulation."

Fever

When people get sick, they often run a fever. Fever is an elevated temperature. Usually a "normal" temperature is considered to be 98.6° Fahrenheit (F) or 37° centigrade (C). However, it is common for some people to have their normal temperature slightly above or below 98.6° F. Temperatures also normally run higher in the afternoon and early evening than in the morning. There is no absolute normal. Learn what yours is. A fever is generally considered an elevation in temperature greater than 1.5 to 2° F or more than 0.8° C.

Your SCI may have affected your body's ability to regulate your temperature. Your body may now be very sensitive to the air temperature. After sitting in the hot sun for several hours, your body temperature may go up even though you are not sick. You may actually have a fever if your temperature rises to over 100° F.

An increased temperature is likely to make you sweat more. The additional moisture can cause your skin to be more likely to break down. It also increases your tissue's need for oxygen and nutrients, because your body is working harder to make you well again.

Solutions

1. Carry a spray bottle of water to mist yourself if you will be out in hot weather for extended times.
2. Wear a broad-brimmed hat.
3. Drink more than your usual liquids to make up for the loss of fluid from fever or heat.

If you have a fever and you think you are sick, call your health-care provider. If you have a fever after you have been in the heat, take two acetaminophen tablets (650 mg total) every four hours. Take a cool bath or sponge yourself with a cool cloth, especially your head, neck, feet, hands, under your arms, and around your groin. If a fever lasts for more than one day, call your health-care provider.

Low Oxygen Levels

You can have a low oxygen problem if you have a lung, heart, or circulation disease. If you are a quadriplegic, your chest muscles are paralyzed and prevent you from taking deep breaths.

Tissues must have oxygen to live. When there is too little oxygen going to your skin, it is more likely to break down.

Solutions

If you have a low-oxygen problem, it is very important for you to read the chapter on "Respiratory Care."

IF YOU SMOKE, STOP!

Follow your health-care providers' recommendations.

Moisture

Anything that causes your skin to be wet or moist, including sweating, urine incontinence, or diarrhea, puts your skin at higher risk for breakdown.

Solutions

1. Keep your skin clean and dry.
2. Pay special attention to cleanliness in areas where you sweat.
3. If you have skin folds, clean and dry under them well.
4. Certain ointments or preparations with lanolin, petroleum jelly, or zinc oxide serve as barriers against moisture. If you develop a reddened area due to moisture, you might try one of these. Like any other reddened area, pay close attention to it. If it does not go away in a week, call your health-care provider.

Underweight

Underweight means being 10% under your ideal body weight. See the "Nutrition" chapter to find your ideal body weight.

Some people who are underweight lack proteins, vitamins, and minerals. Low protein or vitamins can prolong the time it takes to heal a sore if you do develop one. If you are underweight, you may have less soft tissue padding between your sitting bones and skin for protection.

Solutions

Take in extra calories. If you get full quickly, eat more often. Make sure you get plenty of protein-rich food in your diet. If you have limited appetite, eat the nutritious foods first and save the junk food for later. You may also want to take a vitamin supplement. For more information, see the "Nutrition" chapter.

Overweight

Overweight is a relative term. Although there is a large range of weight that is acceptable, we will say that overweight is 10% or more over your ideal body weight. See the "Nutrition" chapter to find your ideal weight.

There are fewer blood vessels in fat tissue. Being overweight causes more pressure on your skin when you sit. This increased weight over pressure points increases the likelihood of skin breakdown.

Being overweight makes it harder for you to move your body around. Transfers are more difficult. Pressure releases may not be as effective.

Solutions

1. Go on a weight-control program. To do so, see or call your dietitian. Read the chapter on "Nutrition" in this handbook.

2. Keep areas between skin folds clean and dry. Inspect your skin twice a day for red areas.

3. Change positions in bed every few hours. Do pressure releases every 15 minutes while sitting. You may need to do a different style of pressure release if you cannot lift your body.

4. Maintain your activity level. Range of motion and being up in your wheelchair are activities. Your physical therapy or recreation therapist will have ideas for including aerobic exercise into your routine.

Peripheral Vascular Disease (PVD)

This is a term that means *atherosclerosis (ATH-ear-o-sclurr-O-siss)*, or hardening of the arteries of the arms or legs (almost always the legs). This affects your circulation. It can be caused by diabetes, smoking, high blood pressure, and elevated *cholesterol (kol-EST-er-all)*.

If the blood vessels are narrow, it is hard to get enough blood to the tissues. This increases the chance of the skin's breaking down by decreasing its oxygen and nutrient supplies.

Solutions

1. *IF YOU SMOKE, STOP!*

2. If you have diabetes, try to keep your blood sugar in control.

3. Keep your feet and legs warm. If your feet and legs are warm, the blood vessels will be as open as possible. If they are cold, the blood vessels will get smaller, which will make the problem worse.

4. Keep your feet and legs very clean. Inspect them daily for sores or reddened areas. If you do get a sore that does not heal within a week, call your health-care provider.

Scar Tissue

A scar is any area of your skin where there was a break or cut in it and a mark, or scar, has formed. Scar tissue has fewer blood vessels and is less elastic than normal skin. It cannot withstand the same amount of pressure and will be more likely to break down.

Solutions

1. Do careful skin inspections over areas with scars.

2. Not all scars will turn red as the first sign of a problem; they may get white and feel hard to the touch. If the scar area starts getting reddened or becomes whiter for a long period, try to stay off it.

Smoking

The nicotine in cigarettes causes the blood vessels to constrict (get small). Smaller blood vessels decrease the amount of blood, oxygen, and nutrients that get to the tissues of the body. This includes the skin. The lack of oxygen and nutrients increases the likelihood of skin breakdown. In addition, hot ashes can fall on your skin and burn you.

Solutions

1. The only way to prevent the effects of nicotine is to stop smoking. Stop-smoking classes are available. Contact your health-care provider.
2. Use cigarette holders if you have impaired use of your hands.
3. Knock the ashes off into an ashtray frequently.
4. Hold the cigarette away from your body.
5. Do not smoke in bed.
6. Wear a fire-retardant cloth on your lap to keep ashes from burning you and your clothes.
7. Install and maintain a smoke alarm in your home.

Sun

Your spinal cord injury has not changed your sensitivity to sunburn.

Solutions

1. Use an SPF #15 or #25 sunscreen.
2. To avoid burns, check sun-heated plastic, vinyl, or metal surfaces before you put any part of your body on them.

TROUBLESHOOTING FOR YOUR SKIN

Table 2.B provides you with a comprehensive look at skin problems that may occur. This table includes a description of what you might see and what you can do to try to solve the problem.

RESOURCES

Publications

Preventing Pressure Ulcers: A Patient's Guide

Treating Pressure Sores: A Consumer's Guide

Purchase:
AHRQ Publications Clearinghouse
P.O. Box 8547
Silver Spring, MD 20907-8547
(800) 358-9295; (888) 586-6340 TDD
Download:
www.ahcpr.gov/news/pubcat/c_title1.htm

Web Sites

www.healthpages.org/AHP/LIBRARY/ HLTHTOP/MISC/bedsore.htm
A web site dedicated to preventing pressure ulcers.

www.woundcarenet.com/
The on-line skin and wound care resource from the publisher of *Advances in Skin & Wound Care* and the joint sponsor of the annual Clinical Symposium on Advances in Skin & Wound Care.

Organizations

Wound, Ostomy and Continence Nurses Society (WOCN)
www.wocn.org

An association of ET nurses, WOGN is a professional nursing society that supports its members by promoting educational, clinical, and research opportunities to advance the practice and guide the delivery of expert health care.

The National Decubitus Foundation
www.decubitus.org

The goals of the organization are to increase public awareness in the areas of education, research, and advocacy for the proper care of individuals with decubitus ulcers.

TABLE 2.B. Troubleshooting for Your Skin

Let your spasticity be a clue to your health. If it gets worse, look for a problem. An example is spasticity that gets worse when you have a urinary tract infection. Any of the following skin problems can cause increased spasticity of your arms or legs.

PROBLEM	WHAT YOU SEE	WHAT YOU DO
Blister	Watery or bloody liquid (fluid) that can be seen under the skin	Do not pop. Keep pressure off of it. If caused by heat, apply cold water soaks immediately. Cover with dry bandage. Phone health-care provider.
Boils	A reddened, tender swelling containing clear fluid.	Do not pop. Wash with mild soap twice a day. Phone health-care provider.
Bruise	A blotchy, bluish-green discoloration of the skin.	Cold compress initially. Keep pressure off bruise until cleared.
Burn	Reddened or blistered skin caused by heat. May be an open sore.	Apply cold water soaks immediately, then keep dry. Do not pop blisters. Do not use ice. Cover with dry bandage. Phone health-care provider.
Frostbite	Whitened or bluish-black numb skin (usually nose, ears, fingers, toes) as a result of exposure to cold.	Gradually and gently rewarm. Cool, then lukewarm water may be used to rewarm frozen parts. Do NOT use hot water bottles or other heat sources. Do NOT rub or massage. Phone health-care provider.
Groin Rash	Reddened area in groin and found in creases and/or all over groin and penis. May be moist and/or pimply.	Wash with mild soap and water 2-3 times a day. Rinse and dry well. Spread legs to air dry. If not better in 2-3 days, phone health-care provider.
Ingrown Toenail	Reddened area around toenail, may have pus when pressed. Nail may be cutting into skin.	Soak in soapy water, wash foot well, rinse, and dry. Put small piece of cotton under nail to keep edge of nail away from skin. Change cotton daily. Cut toenail straight across. If it does not begin to heal in 2-3 days, phone health-care provider.
Open Cut and Sores	A wound in or through the skin.	Apply pressure if bleeding. Wash with water or saline, rinse, and dry. Apply bandage. Keep pressure off of sore. Phone health-care provider if in area you have no feeling or if redness or pus is present.
Pimples	Small reddened sores with a pus head on the skin.	Do NOT pop. Wash twice a day with mild soap. Dry skin well. If pimples do not dry up, phone health-care provider.
Pressure Sores	A sore usually over a bony area. See Pressure Sore Chapter.	Wash with water or saline, rinse, and dry. Apply bandage if sore is open. Keep all pressure off the sore. Phone health-care provider.
Red Area	Red skin that does not fade in 15 minutes. Does not blanch (turn white when pressure is put on it).	Do not put pressure on the area until the redness fades completely. May take days.
Sunburn	Dry, red skin with or without blisters, fever.	Apply cold water soaks to skin for comfort, then soothing creams. Do NOT pop blisters. Cover blisters with bandage. If fever persists, call health-care provider.
Swelling	An abnormal enlargement or increase in size of body part, usually on arms or legs. May also have color change—red or black and blue.	Elevate the swollen part and wear your compressive hose. See the chapters on "Nerve, Muscles & Bones" and "Circulation." If swelling is not even from one side to the other, call your health-care provider.

Circulatory System | *Chapter* 3

The circulatory system distributes nutrients from food and oxygen from your lungs throughout your body. Your circulatory system is made up of your *heart, arteries, capillaries (CAP-ill-air-ees), and veins.* Blood travels throughout your body by way of this system. *(See figure 3.1.)*

There are several specific changes that affect your circulation after an SCI. After a

FIGURE 3.1. Circulatory System

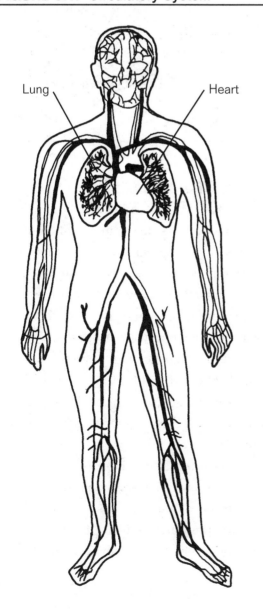

Lung

Heart

quick look at the basics, we will describe these changes to help you recognize if there may be a problem.

HOW THE CIRCULATORY SYSTEM WORKS

Getting blood to every cell in your body is the job of your heart. It acts as a pump, sending fluid through a system of tubes or blood vessels. Blood comes into the *right side of your heart* from your body and is pumped out to the tissues of the lungs, where it picks up oxygen. (*Please note:* Blood does not go into the air space of your lungs. Blood runs throughout the walls of your lungs like wiring in the walls of your house.)

After leaving the lungs, it then returns to the *left side of the heart* and is pumped out into the arteries. The arteries carry it to the *capillaries*. These tiny blood vessels run throughout the tissues of your body. There they deliver oxygen, pick up waste products, and distribute nutrients as needed.

The blood leaves the capillaries by way of the *veins*. Veins return blood to the *right side of your heart*, where the whole cycle begins again. *(See figure 3.2.)*

Blood Pressure and How It's Regulated

Blood pressure is a measure of the force with which your blood goes through your blood vessels. It is basically determined by two things:

1. How well your heart can pump blood out.

2. How much tension there is in your arteries.

FIGURE 3.2. How Circulation Works

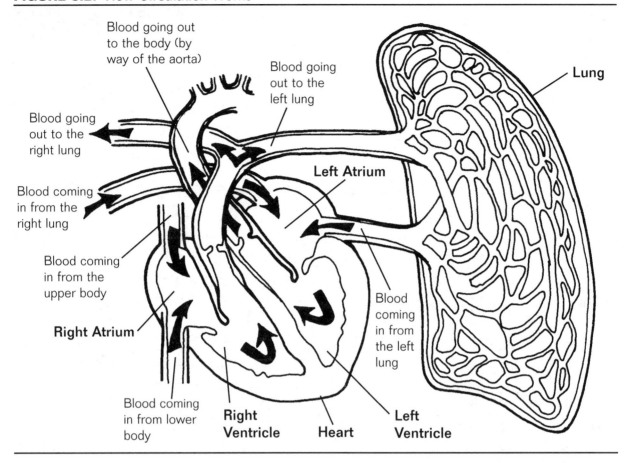

Blood going out to the body (by way of the aorta)

Blood going out to the left lung

Blood going out to the right lung

Blood coming in from the right lung

Blood coming in from the upper body

Right Atrium

Blood coming in from lower body

Right Ventricle

Heart

Left Ventricle

Blood coming in from the left lung

Left Atrium

Lung

There is a wide range of blood pressures that are considered normal. *A stable blood pressure* is one that stays within a consistent range.

Your *nervous system* controls the diameter of your blood vessels. The diameter is always adjusting in size depending on your body position and level of activity. This helps keep your blood pressure stable. For example, when you move from sitting to standing, the blood vessels in your legs narrow to stabilize blood pressure. If this did not occur, blood would stay in your legs rather than return to your heart. This pooling of blood in your legs would cause your blood pressure to lower.

HOW SCI AFFECTS YOUR CIRCULATION

The major effects that your spinal cord injury has on your circulation are changes in your blood pressure and in how your blood moves from your body back to your heart. How well your heart pumps is not affected by SCI but the tension in your arteries is.

As mentioned above, your nervous system plays a part in adjusting the diameter of your arteries. So, the arteries in the parts of your body affected by your injury will also be affected.

A narrow artery raises blood pressure, while a wider artery lowers the pressure. Think in terms of a garden hose. At the tap, you turn on the water and let it flow at a steady rate. Depending on how you use the nozzle, you can close it down and increase the resistance, sending less water through in a high-powered, direct stream. You can also open the nozzle all the way and decrease the resistance, which will give you a lot of water in a relaxed spray with no strong power behind it.

Increasing the blood pressure is like closing down the nozzle. Lowering the blood pressure is like opening up the nozzle so that the power behind the water is little more than what originally comes from the tap. By closing down the nozzle just enough, you can take the original power behind the water, force it through a smaller space, and increase the power and speed at which it comes out. You can then shoot down your neighbor's prize roses at 40 paces!

In the same way, a *stable blood pressure* is high enough to circulate nutrients and oxygen to your body quickly and efficiently but not so high as to cause you problems.

After SCI, your arteries tend to stay wide *(dilated)*. They can't get as narrow *(constricted)* as they did before your SCI. The result is that your blood pressure stabilizes at a lower level than it was before your injury.

Usually, the *action of your muscles,* flexing and relaxing either voluntarily or during spasticity, helps keep your blood moving. The muscles affected by your injury can't do this any more, although spasticity can help somewhat.

These changes in your circulation after SCI tend to increase your risk for developing the following conditions:

1. Edema (swelling)
2. Thrombus/pulmonary embolus (blood clots)
3. Orthostatic hypotension (low blood pressure when you sit up)
4. Decreased heart rate

Edema (swelling)

Depending on the level of your injury, your legs and perhaps your hands may swell. Swelling occurs when fluid leaves your blood vessels and goes into the spaces between tissue cells. This swelling is called "*dependent edema.*" (Dependent refers to any area that is below the level of your heart.) This edema is caused by muscle weakness in your legs or arms, because muscle action and movement normally help return blood to your heart. If the blood returns to the heart too slowly, more fluid will leak out of the blood and into the spaces between tissue cells.

To prevent your legs from swelling, you can do the following:

1. *Wear stockings routinely.* These are tight elastic stockings and should generally come up to the top of your thigh. They help in returning blood to your heart and keeping it from pooling in your legs.

2. *Do your range-of-motion exercises every day,* and make sure that you move your legs from one position to another every two to three hours.

If the swelling is only in one of your legs, see the next section because you may have a blood clot in your leg! If both your legs swell, try these tips for decreasing edema:

1. *Do more range-of-motion exercises. Do them routinely* or get someone else to do it for you.

2. *Elevate your legs* to or above the level of your heart for 10 to 15 minutes. Do this four to five times a day. Here are some ways to do this:

   • Lie down and place pillows under your feet and calves and/or under your hands and arms.

- Move your wheelchair close to your bed and place your feet and legs on the bed. *LOCK YOUR WHEELCHAIR FIRST!*

- Sit on a couch or an overstuffed chair and place your feet and legs on your wheelchair.

- Sleep with your legs slightly elevated.

3. *Make sure you wear your compressive stockings* while you are awake and up in your chair.

4. *If the swelling continues* in your legs for more than one week despite your efforts to treat it or if you notice a sudden increase in swelling, call your physician at the SCI center or in your community.

Thrombus *or* DVT (blood clot)

Blood clots in either your legs or your lungs can be a serious medical problem. Blood has a tendency to clot when it does not move at its regular, steady pace. The same lack of muscle pumping action in your legs that causes swelling slows the blood and allows clots to form. Blood clots begin in veins, especially those in your legs. If it's in one of the veins deep inside your leg, it is called a "DVT" *(deep vein thrombus)*. *(See figure 3.3.)* A blood clot in the leg veins can break free and travel to other parts of your body. A clot that stays in one place is a thrombus (plural = thrombi). A clot that has broken free is called an *embolus* (plural = emboli).

The most common place for an embolus to go is the lung. This is called a *"pulmonary embolus."* Because *this is an emergency*, the health-care staff will pay a lot of attention to you to help prevent this complication. You will need to learn how to decrease the chance of this happening.

FIGURE 3.3. Thrombus in Leg

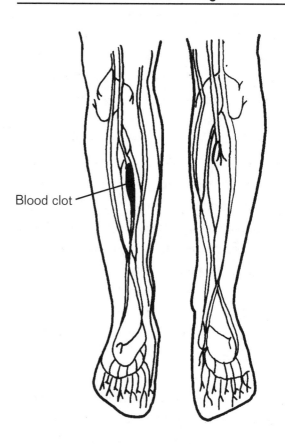

Blood clot

Blood clots are very common after SCI. Your risk is greatest during the first few months after injury. Blood clots are common when activity is decreased, since the blood moves slowly through the leg veins. Surgery and injury to the legs can also increase the risk of blood clots. Eventually the risk of blood clots decreases, but it is always more of a risk than for people without SCI.

Some conditions increase the risk of blood clots. People can't avoid some of these things, such as having cancer or broken leg bones, needing surgery, being older, or having heart failure. You should try to avoid the following risky conditions: weight gain, cigarette smoking, dehydration, and unnecessary inactivity. Pregnancy also increases the risk of blood clots, so women who want to get pregnant need to be careful to watch for symptoms of blood clots. Finally, if you've already had a blood clot, it's more likely that you will have another.

Since blood clots are so common, your doctors often use drugs and other treatments to try and prevent them. First, the same things used to treat swelling (listed above) are started. Your doctor might also put you on medication that will decrease clot formation. These drugs are commonly known as "blood thinners" or *anticoagulants (ANN-tie-co-AGG-you-lance)*. The most common type of drug used to prevent blood clots is called heparin. There are different types of heparin that have names like enoxaparin, Lovenox, and low molecular weight heparin. Sometimes doctors also use plastic air pumps on the legs to prevent blood clots. The part that goes around the leg inflates with air. This pushes the blood out of the legs and back toward the heart. These treatments decrease the risk of blood clots, but some people will get blood clots even if they receive the drugs and other treatments.

Some common signs and symptoms of a clot in your leg include:

1. One calf or thigh feels warmer than the other. It may also be red.

2. One calf or thigh is more swollen than the other. A simple way to see if there might be swelling is to measure the size of both calves or thighs. A clot can develop and cause the leg to swell quickly. This is why, in the early stages after your injury, the nursing staff measure the size of your calves and thighs. You may wish to continue this practice on a weekly basis at home.

3. One leg may be painful, tender, or feel heavy. However, you may not have normal feeling in your legs, so you may not feel anything.

Often when there is a blood clot, you can not tell you have one and neither can your doctors without doing special tests.

What to Do if You Think You Have One

1. If one calf or thigh becomes larger than the other:
   - *DO NOT* increase your activity level.
   - *DO NOT* do range-of-motion exercises.
   - *DO NOT* move the leg. Increasing your activity may cause the clot to break loose.

2. Put yourself to bed and call your physician or nurse at the spinal cord center to get further instructions. If you do have a clot in your leg, treatment will be geared toward preventing it from breaking free and moving to your lungs.

3. Most people with a blood clot must take anticoagulants for three to six months after the clot is discovered.

How to Tell if You May Have a Pulmonary Embolus (Blood Clot in the Lung)

You may feel one or all of the following:

1. A sudden shortness of breath. It may be accompanied by a feeling of tightness in your chest.

2. Pain in your side, chest, or back. The pain is usually worse when you breathe in and lets up when you breathe out.

3. A sudden development of a new cough. This cough is often associated with sputum or phlegm that may be slightly pink or red.

Prevention

Prevention is extremely important, because a pulmonary embolus can be life-threatening. Since most pulmonary emboli are caused by clots in the legs, the way to prevent them is to follow the prevention methods given to you under "prevention of blood clots."

What to Do if You Think You Have a Pulmonary Embolus

1. *CALL 911. A pulmonary embolus is an emergency!*

2. *Also call your spinal cord center physician* or your local physician immediately.

3. *If you feel short of breath*, sit up in a chair; this sometimes helps.

4. *This problem needs to be treated in a hospital* where further tests and treatments can be performed.

Treatment of Blood Clots

If you get a blood clot in your leg, or if it goes into the lung, you will usually receive blood thinners to help your body dissolve the blood clot. The most common blood thinners are heparin and warfarin (Coumadin). The main side effect of these drugs is bleeding. Bleeding can be minor, like a nosebleed, or serious, like a bleeding stomach ulcer. Because of these risks, people on blood thinners need close medical follow-up. Sometimes frequent blood tests are needed to make sure you are receiving the right dose of the blood thinners. Some of these medicines can interact with other drugs, or even with food. You should ask for information about these interactions if you need to take blood thinners after leaving the hospital. Usually a pharmacist will discuss this with you if you need blood thinners.

Orthostatic Hypotension

Your blood pressure may be lower after an SCI, because your blood vessels cannot constrict to help keep it at a higher level. Most people get used to a lower blood pressure and do not have problems from it.

However, when you sit up with your legs down or when you stand up, your blood pressure may drop even lower. This happens because blood tends to collect (pool) in the veins of your legs and feet instead of being pushed back to the heart. If your blood pressure drops when you are upright, it is called *orthostatic hypotension*. Orthostatic means "changing positions," and hypotension refers to lower blood pressure.

Lower blood pressure can decrease the amount of blood to your brain. This makes you feel lightheaded or dizzy when you change positions. This can be a big problem soon after your SCI when you first get out of bed. Fortunately, this problem usually improves with time in most people.

Preventing Lightheadness or Dizziness

1. When you get up from a lying position, do it in steps:
   - Sit up slowly.
   - Rest for a few minutes.
   - Move your legs to a lower position.
   - Continue your activities.

2. Do not change positions quickly. Take your time.

3. Wear your compressive stockings and abdominal binder (if prescribed), because they help blood get back to your heart and help prevent blood from collecting in your legs.

If you have a continuing problem with dizziness, you can try the following:

1. Make sure that you are taking in enough fluids in your diet.

2. If you continue to feel dizzy or lightheaded despite following all the tips outlined above, call your SCI clinic physician or nurse. You may need to be put on medications to increase your blood pressure for a while.

Your blood pressure can go so low that not enough blood gets to your brain and you pass out, or faint. Fainting should not cause problems if it happens once in a while. If it does occur more often, you need to be treated to prevent it.

If You Faint or Feel Dizzy

1. Your family or attendant should lie you down and elevate your legs to above the level of your heart.

2. If you are in your wheelchair, someone can just tilt the wheelchair backwards about 45 degrees. Be sure to lock your brakes first.

Decreased Heart Rate

After an injury to the spinal cord, your heart rate will tend to be slower. The same part of the nervous system that is responsible for increasing your blood pressure is also responsible for increasing your heart rate. This ability may be lost if your injury is *above the mid-thoracic level.* If you cannot raise

your heart rate when you need to, such as when exercising, you may have the same feelings of dizziness and lightheadedness that were mentioned in the section on orthostatic hypotension.

What Will You Feel if You Have Decreased Heart Rate?

Most people don't feel any differently with decreased heart rate. Some people, though, may feel dizziness and lightheadedness if their heart rate drops below 50 beats per minute.

If you feel lightheaded or dizzy, call your SCI clinic for further instructions.

It's a good idea to memorize your usual blood pressure and heart rate. That way, if you are treated by different doctors who don't have your medical records, you can tell them what is a normal blood pressure and heart rate for you. Otherwise, they may think you have a new medical problem causing low blood pressure or pulse.

Breathing is the voluntary and involuntary movement of air, in and out, either your nose or your mouth. The two purposes of breathing are:

- To get *oxygen* (O_2) to your tissues for survival, and
- To remove the waste product of the cells, *carbon dioxide* (CO_2).

The exchange of gases is the job of your *lungs*. In the lungs, oxygen (O_2) tubes come down from your windpipe and branch from your neck down into your chest like a tree growing upside down. *(See figure 4.1.)*

These tubes keep branching until they are very tiny. At the very end of the smallest branch are air sacs that look like little clusters of balloons. These balloons are located next to the blood vessels in the walls of your lungs. Because of the way your lungs are built, when you inhale, air is sucked into the balloons to fully inflate them. The oxygen is then passed to red blood cells in the blood vessels to be carried to the rest of the body by way of your heart. The carbon dioxide (CO_2) waste in your blood is passed into your lungs so that when you breathe out, you get rid of it. See the chapter on the "Circulatory System" for more information.

Breathing out generally takes no effort or energy. Breathing in does require energy. The faster you breathe, the more energy it takes. Breathing in requires many different muscles. *(See table 4.A.)*

KEEPING YOUR LUNGS HEALTHY

1. *Stop smoking.* Smoking increases your secretions and likelihood of getting infections. It prevents the lung's natural action to get rid of pollutants.

2. *Do breathing exercises on a regular basis* if you have a cervical or high-thoracic level of injury. If you have an incentive spirometer, use it at least two or three times a day. If you don't have one, take as deep a breath in as you can two or three times a day. Hold it for a count of three, then push all the air out. Do that 5 to 10 times each session.

   You may also learn something called "frog breathing" to help you increase the amount of air in your lungs. It is a type of breathing exercise that you can learn

FIGURE 4.1. The Respiratory System

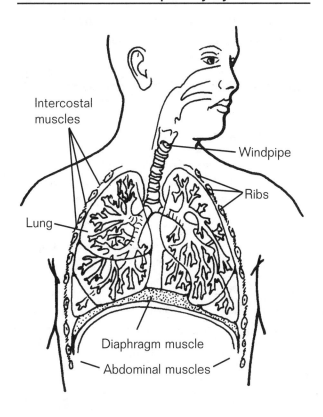

Intercostal muscles

Windpipe

Ribs

Lung

Diaphragm muscle

Abdominal muscles

TABLE 4.A. Some of the Muscles Used in Breathing

RESPIRATORY MUSCLES	FUNCTION	SPINAL CORD INJURY LEVEL AND ITS EFFECT ON BREATHING
Diaphragm	The main muscle of breathing. It is found just underneath your lungs.	An injury above C5 may require the use of a breathing machine for a while or permanently, because the diaphragm and most other muscles may not work.*
Intercostals	These muscles run in between your ribs. They are used in coughing and deep breathing.	An injury above T1 will reduce the strength of these muscles, but diaphragm and neck muscles can assist breathing.
Abdominals	These muscles help you in coughing. They run between your ribs and your hips.	An injury above T12 will reduce the strength of these muscles, but intercostals, diaphragm, and neck muscles can assist.

*If you use a breathing machine, you will get special training in its use.

with practice. This is taught by speech therapists to patients who need this type of exercise.

3. *Try to stay away from known pollutants*, such as smoke, dusts, and dangerous chemicals.

4. *If you get a cold or sore throat*, do more breathing exercises. If you have a cold, perform quad coughing two or three times a day. This should help prevent the build up of secretions and the risk of a *pneumonia (new-MOAN-yah). Take it seriously.* If a cold or sore throat does not go away in a week to 10 days, contact your SCI clinic or your doctor for further instructions.

5. The use of an abdominal binder can increase respiratory capacity by substituting for a paralyzed abdominal wall.

RESPIRATORY PROBLEMS

Respiratory problems can be caused by many things, but by far the most common problem is an infection, such as pneumonia. Other problems can cause you to feel the same way.

You may experience any or all of the following symptoms of infection:

1. Increased shortness of breath.

2. Rapid breathing.

3. Increased congestion or secretions from your lungs.

4. Lower reading of air flow through your incentive spirometer.

5. Early morning headache, fever, or unusual drowsiness.

Treating Respiratory Problems

1. *Increase the number* of times you do your breathing exercises. Do them every two hours.

2. *Quad coughing* can be done to increase the effectiveness of your cough. This is done by having someone else push over your abdomen at the same time you cough. *NOTE: Do not attempt this if it has never been demonstrated to you.* Self-assisted coughing can be done by bracing your arms, leaning forward, and putting pressure on the abdomen.

3. *Change your position* more frequently by moving from sitting to lying and by turning from side to side. This will change the areas of your lungs that get air and will help you keep all areas of your lungs working.

4. *Do postural drainage* after your breathing exercises, whenever time and place allow, *but only if you have been taught how to do it properly*. Putting your head and chest down allows secretions to drain by gravity toward the upper lung. They can then be coughed up more easily.

5. *Chest percussion* can also be done while you are lying head down. Get someone to clap their hands on your chest. This also aids in removal of secretions. You must be taught how to do this properly.

6. *Consider taking a warm (not hot!) bath or shower*. This warms and humidifies the air with steam. Steam can help liquefy secretions so that they become easier to cough up. Do this once or twice a day, then cough.

7. Increase fluids to thin your secretions, which will make it easier to cough these secretions up.

If your symptoms do not go away in 5 to 10 days and your treatments don't seem to help, call the SCI clinic.

If your symptoms are getting worse or if you have a fever, call your SCI clinic or local doctor.

Some respiratory infections may need *antibiotics* to kill bacteria or medications to help you breathe better and easier. Those decisions may require that the SCI clinic staff see you. Serious breathing problems may need to be treated in the hospital. Fever, chills, and cough that is associated with shortness of breath should be evaluated by SCI clinic staff.

Sleep Apnea

What is sleep apnea?

People with sleep apnea stop breathing for at least 10 seconds at a time while they are sleeping. These short stops in breathing can happen up to 400 times every night. The periods of not breathing can make you wake up from deep sleep. If you're waking up so often all night long, you aren't getting enough rest from your sleep.

How do you know if you have sleep apnea?

- Your doctor can diagnose sleep apnea.

- The person you sleep with or your caretaker may notice heavy snoring or long pauses in your breathing during sleep.

- You may notice daytime sleepiness (falling asleep at work, while driving, or when talking) and irritability or fatigue.

- You may also notice that you have morning headaches, forgetfulness, mood changes, and a decreased interest in sex.

There are steps that may help people with sleep apnea to sleep better.

- Stop all use of alcohol or sleep medicines.

- If you are overweight, lose weight.

- Sleep on your side instead of on your back.

If you still have problems, you can wear a special mask over your nose and mouth while you are sleeping. The flow of the air from the machine will keep your airway open by adding pressure to the air you breathe. In a very few cases, surgery is necessary to remove tonsils or extra tissue in the throat.

You may request a sleep apnea consultation from your physician.

Range of Motion | Chapter 5

Your body is made up of a series of bones, muscles, and *joints*. The joints are bone junctions. The purpose of the joints is to provide motion within your body and to support or bear weight. Joints are surrounded by muscles, tendons, ligaments, and a joint capsule that provide stability to the joint. The muscles that cross a joint create movement of the bones on either side.

The range of motion (or number of degrees of motion) at a joint is determined by the tightness of the ligaments, tendons, muscles, and joint capsule surrounding that joint—the looser or more flexible the structures, the more movement. The tighter the structures, the less movement.

Prolonged tightness of a joint and the structures around it can lead to permanently shortened range of motion. This is called a *contracture (con-TRACK-churr)*. The treatment for contractures includes static stretching (prolonged positioning and stretching of the muscles and joints) and heat treatments. Contracture may require extensive surgical procedures. Contractures are at the least disfiguring and cause other problems, such as pressure sores and loss of ability to perform physical activities. They significantly interfere with hygiene. The best plan is to avoid contractures. See the chapter on "Nerves, Muscles & Bones."

Generally, the everyday movements of a person are enough to keep his or her joints and the muscles that cross them loose and flexible. The weakness caused by your spinal cord injury may interfere with the full range of motion of your joints. Because of this weakness and the resulting loss of movement, it is necessary to find some other means to stretch your muscles and to maintain the flexibility of the joints and surrounding structures.

Loss of motion will often show up in predictable patterns after a spinal cord injury. Sitting in a wheelchair shortens the muscles that cross the front of the hips and the back of the knees. If you are not sitting in a fully erect posture, you can also see tightness in the front of the shoulders and neck from a forward slouched posture. Blankets can also cause the toes to point downward while you are lying in bed, which can shorten the muscle at the back of the ankle.

It is important to stretch these muscles to counter the shortening caused by positioning or the tightness can become fixed (contracture) and limit your ability to move. Loss of motion affects you and your body in many ways. Tightness of your joints, whether it is in your hips, knees, or shoulders, often limits the positions into which you can move your body. This limits the activities you can do for yourself. In addition to positional shortening, use of a manual wheelchair promotes strengthening and tightness in the anterior muscles of the shoulder. This can lead to a rounded shoulder posture. Careful stretching of the anterior muscles and strengthening of the posterior muscles can improve the muscle balance around the shoulder.

Tightness of your trunk and legs may also affect your sitting or standing posture, especially when there is more tightness on one side of your body than the other. This can lead to a curving or twisting of your back and throw off the balance of your body. Decreased range of motion of your arms, legs, and trunk tends to increase pressure at localized points rather than allowing pressure to be evenly distributed. This localization of pressure significantly increases your risks of skin breakdown. Optimal seated posture is critical to maintaining healthy skin and pain-free shoulders.

Loss of motion in your hips can also interfere with the cleansing of your groin and especially interfere with positioning your legs during sex. Maintaining the flexibility of your muscles also tends to decrease spasticity.

Your physical and occupational therapists will instruct you in how to do your own range of motion exercises. A program will be designed specifically for you and your individual needs. If you are not able to do your exercises by yourself, you will be taught how to instruct others to do the exercises for you. Remember, even if you are unable to do the exercises yourself, you are still responsible for your own body and what is done to it.

In some cases, especially with hands, your therapists may allow for a certain amount of tightening in some of the tendons of your hands and wrists. This selective shortening can sometimes increase the function of your hands through an action called *tenodesis (ten-oh-DEE-siss)*.

As important as range of motion is, and it is very important, so is having time for things you enjoy. If you have a high cervical spinal cord injury, you may need assistance with many daily tasks. It is very important that you spend a realistic amount of time for range of motion exercises. Ask your therapist which exercises are the most critical for you. Ask your therapist how you can incorporate the exercises into dressing or bathing activities. It may also be possible to design a program with exercises that rotate each day so that you are

spending a maximum of thirty minutes a day on range of motion.

On the other hand, if you have a low lumbar spinal cord injury you have a different problem. Your muscles have no contractile element (no "pull back") so your problem is getting too loose. Ask your therapist to show you clear and specific stopping points for all motions of your legs.

Everyone with a spinal cord injury should pay special attention to not allowing the muscle in front of the hip (the hip flexor) to get tight. This is a big strong muscle and once tight makes for many positioning problems in bed, in a wheelchair, or standing. The best recommendation for this muscle is lying on your stomach (prone lying) at least twice a day. It is important to start this early after your SCI because once this muscle is tight, lying on your stomach will just arch your back and not really stretch the hip flexor.

SELF-STRETCHING

Self passive range-of-motion (PROM) technique can and should be an efficient package.

First lie on your stomach (prone): key is to have your feet off the end of the bed. This will help keep your hips down on the bed. Next move up on to your elbows but keep your belly button on the bed surface. You should stay here for about 5 minutes or more if you have a lot of spasticity. It is a good way to get some reading done. Now move up into long sitting. Bring one knee up toward your chest and then place it so that leg is crossed over the other, with your foot just above your other knee. In this position you can do a number of stretches. First stretch the top ankle: reach to the foot and stretch into dorsiflexion (pull the foot up). This works best if you place the bottom of your foot against your forearm to push up while you are pushing down on your knee with your opposite hand. The "hug" position also stabilizes you for the stretch. Now reach for your other foot, the one on the straight leg. Reach with the same side arm by rotation of the body and chest elevation (translates to anterior pelvic tilt) this will provide a hamstring stretch at the same time you stretch the ankle. Switch legs and repeat.

In doing your range-of-motion exercises, allow time for your muscles and other structures to loosen and stretch. We recommend that you hold the position for a slow count of 10. When you are moving your body, move slowly and smoothly. Then, as you hold the position, maintain a firm but gentle pressure. Do not bounce your body, as this tends to encourage spastic muscles to tighten.

Some Important Points to Remember

1. *NEVER use excessive force when stretching.* All that is required is enough force to allow the muscle fibers to lengthen (stretch). Excessive force can result in fractures, torn or pulled muscles, or dislocated joints.

2. *Hold the position still*, rather than bouncing, especially if you have spasticity. This allows your muscle fibers to relax and stretch. Bouncing increases the tension in muscles.

3. *A good time to do your stretching program* is in the morning or in the evening when you do your skin inspection.

EXERCISES FOR ASSISTED RANGE OF MOTION

The following series of range of motion exercises use the "SAM" format, outlining the correct motions and body positioning required

to perform them safely. Please remind your attendants to use careful movements and not stretch out or hurt their backs!

SAM:

S: Your **STARTING** position.

A: Your **ATTENDANT'S** action/position.

M: The actual **MOVEMENT**.

Trunk Rotation

S: Lying on your back with your knees bent to your chest.

A: Kneeling at your feet with both hands placed on your knees.

M: Rotate your knees and hips to one side; bring them as close to the bed as they will go; keep your shoulders flat on the bed. Your attendant may need to put one hand on your opposite shoulder to hold it down.

Trunk Bending

S: Lying on your back with your legs together and your knees bent toward your chest.

A: Kneeling at your feet with both hands placed on your knees.

M: Bend your knees to your chest, stretching your back muscles.

Hip Abduction with Knees Bent

S: Lying on your back with your legs bent.

A: Kneeling with your feet between attendant's knees to hold them in place, each hand placed on your knee.

M: Spread your knees apart, and down towards the bed, applying a firm (but not heavy) pressure.

Hip Extension

S: Lying on your side, not leaning forward or back, with your upper leg slightly bent.

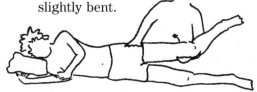

A: Kneeling behind you, one arm cupping under your knee with your calf resting on his or her forearm, and the other hand holding your pelvis in place.

M: Pull your leg straight backwards toward your attendant.

Stretches (Hip Flexion & Extension)

S: Lying on your back with your toes pointing toward the ceiling, one knee bent toward your chest.

A: One hand placed on your bent knee, the other hand placed just above the knee of your straight leg.

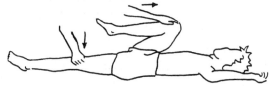

M: Bend your bent leg further toward your chest, keeping your other leg straight on the bed.

Leg Rotation

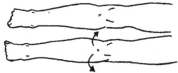

S: Lying in bed, your legs straight and relaxed.

A: Hands placed on top of your thigh, or one hand on top of your thigh, the other underneath your thigh.

M: Roll your knee in and out. Do not have your attendant's hands placed below your knee or there will be excessive stress to your knee.

Heel Cord (Gastroc/Soleus)

S: Lying on your back with your knees straight.

A: One hand cups the inside of your heel, with the forearm pressed up against the ball of your foot.

M: Keeping your knee straight, pull down at your heel and press up with the forearm, bending your foot toward your knee.

Straight Leg Raise (SLR)

S: Lying on your back with your legs straight and slightly apart.

A: Two positions possible:

1. Kneeling between your legs, with one hand cupping your heel while the other hand is holding the knee of the same leg. The attendant's knee may be resting lightly on your other thigh to stabilize your leg on the bed.

2. Kneeling between your legs, with your heel cord resting on the attendant's shoulder. One of the attendant's hands should be placed on that knee to keep

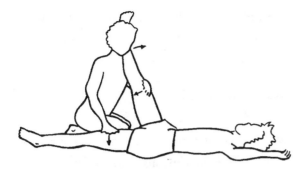

it straight, the other hand should be on your other thigh to stabilize that leg on the bed.

M: Slowly raise your leg up, keeping your knee straight. Do not allow your leg to roll out. When your raised knee begins to bend slightly from the tension, have your attendant lower your leg slightly and hold. Do not move beyond the leg pointing straight up to the ceiling.

Scapular Circumduction

S: Lying on your side with your arm resting on your hip or behind your back.

A: One hand cupping the front of your shoulder, the other placed so the web of the thumb meets with the angle of your shoulder blade.

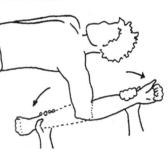

M: Moving both hands circularly in the same direction, roll the shoulder blade slowly in a large circle.

Scapular Protraction

S: Lying on your side with your arm resting on your hip or behind your back.

A: One hand cupping the front of your shoulder, the other placed so that the pinkie side of the attendant's hand is next to your shoulder blade.

M: Applying a firm pressure backwards on your shoulder, slide the other hand under your shoulder blade, lifting away from your back.

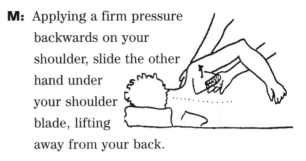

Shoulder Rotation

S: Your arm out from your side at about 45 degrees, your elbow bent 90°.

A: One hand cupping your elbow, the other supporting your wrist and hand.

M: Rotate your hand toward the bed by your pillow, and then toward your hip. Keep your elbow bent at 90°.

Abduction

S: Lying on your back with your arm at your side and your palm up.

A: One hand supporting your hand and wrist, the other cupping your elbow.

M: Bring your arm out to your side up to your head (similar to the movement in jumping jacks).

Forward Flexion

S: Your arm at your side, palm up.

A: One hand supporting your wrist/hand, the other supporting the back of your elbow.

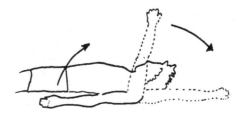

M: Raise your arm up over your head, with your thumbleading, pointing first at the ceiling and finally the wall. Keep the elbow relatively straight.

Shoulder Extension

S: Sitting in your chair or lying on your side in bed.

A: One hand stabilizing your shoulder, the other cupping your arm near your elbow.

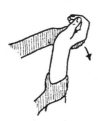

M: Bring your arm back behind you as if you were going to reach into your rear pocket.

Elbow Flexion/Extension

S: Your arm straight at your side, palm up.

A: One hand supporting your wrist and hand, the other stabilizing your upper arm.

M: Straighten your arm to its fullest, then bend your elbow, bringing your hand to your shoulder.

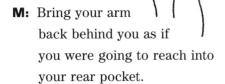

Supination/Pronation

S: Your arm at your side with your elbow bent 90°.

A: Supporting your wrist/hand and stabilizing your arm just above your elbow.

M: Turn your palm up, then turn your palm down.

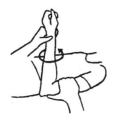 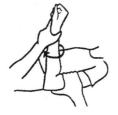

Repeat the above with your elbow straight. You can combine this exercise with the one above (Elbow Flexion/Extension)

Wrist Flexion/Extension

S: Wrist and fingers relaxed.

A: One hand supporting your forearm, the other hand clasping your palm—be certain that your fingers are free to move.

 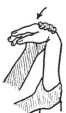

M: Bend your wrist down, allowing your fingers to straighten at will. Bend your wrist up, being certain that your attendant's hand and fingers do not interfere with your fingers' bending.

Wrist Deviation

S: Your wrist in line with your arm, not bent up or down.

A: Supporting your hand, the other stabilizing your forearm.

M: Move your hand side to side, not allowing your wrist to bend up or down.

Finger Flexion

S: Your fingers relaxed, your wrist bent up.

A: Supporting your hand and wrist.

M: Gently bend your fingers toward your palm, being certain to keep your wrist cocked (bent) up.

Finger Extension

S: Wrist and fingers relaxed.

A: One hand supporting your forearm and keeping your wrist bent down, the other hand cupping your finger tips.

M: Keeping your wrist bent down, straighten your fingers. The movement should come from your knuckles and the joints of your fingers, not your wrist.

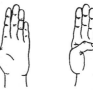

Finger Abduction

S: Wrist straight, fingers and thumb relaxed.

A: Holding adjacent fingers straight.

M: Spread fingers apart.

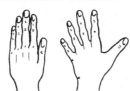

Hand Mobilization

S: Your palm down with your thumb and fingers relaxed.

A: Cupping your hand in both hands, the attendant's right thumb and index finger hold one knuckle while the left thumb and index finger hold the next knuckle over.

M: One hand gently pushes down on the knuckle it is holding while the other hand pushes up. Reverse directions. Move across your hand.

Thumb Abduction/Extension

S: Palm up with your fingers and thumb relaxed.

A: One hand stabilizing your palm, the other grasping your thumb with your attendant's thumb at the base of your thumb.

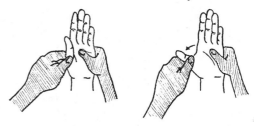

M: Move your thumb out and away from your palm as if you were hitch-hiking.

Thumb Opposition

S: Palm up with your fingers and thumb relaxed.

A: Holding your thumb over your nail.

M: Touch the tip of your thumb to the base of your little finger.

Bladder Management | *Chapter* 6

Before your spinal cord injury, you probably did not pay much attention to your urinary system because urinating occurred so automatically. During the first few months after injury, you and certain members of the spinal cord injury team will be spending what seems like a great deal of time helping you establish and manage your bladder program. Eventually, your bladder program will become quick and routine for you.

THE URINARY SYSTEM

The urinary system consists of the *kidneys*, the *ureters (YURR-ut-airs)*, the *bladder*, and the *urethra (yur-EE-thra)*. *(See figures 6.1 and 6.2.)*

The primary differences between the male and female urinary systems are the length of the urethra and the presence of a prostate in the male. Otherwise, the systems are the same.

The *kidneys* remove waste and excess water from your blood stream and process them into urine. The urine then flows down the *ureters* (which are small tubes) to your *bladder*. The bladder is a muscular sac that stretches to hold urine until you are ready to *void (urinate)*. When voiding occurs, the bladder (also called the *detrusor muscle*) contracts and the sphincter (which is a circular muscle acting as a gate) opens. Urine then passes through the *urethra* and you urinate.

Urination calls for a finely balanced coordination of bladder and sphincter muscles. This coordination involves both voluntary and involuntary (or automatic) control by the nervous system. When the bladder becomes full,

FIGURE 6.1 Male Urinary System

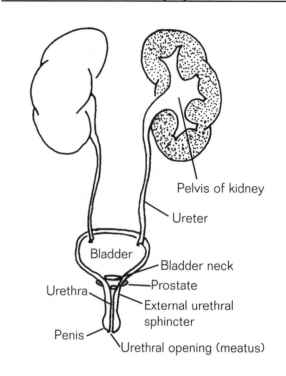

Pelvis of kidney
Ureter
Bladder
Bladder neck
Prostate
Urethra
External urethral sphincter
Penis
Urethral opening (meatus)

FIGURE 6.2 Female Urinary System

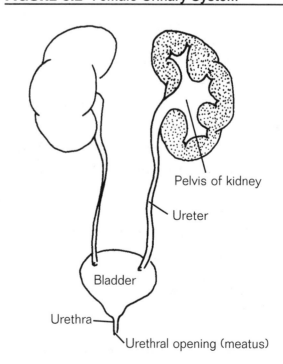

Pelvis of kidney
Ureter
Bladder
Urethra
Urethral opening (meatus)

nerve impulses are sent to the sacral level of the spinal cord, and then sent to your brain to let you know that your bladder is full. At that time, you can decide to either urinate or hold the urine. This is the part under *voluntary control.* If you want to void, the brain will send messages back to the urinary system. The *involuntary* part involves the opening of the sphincter muscle and bladder muscle contraction.

Changes in Bladder Function After SCI

Following SCI, nerve impulses from the bladder can no longer get to and from the brain to let you sense that your bladder is full or to let you void. There are two general kinds of bladder dysfunction that can occur, depending on your level of injury. Because there can be individual variations, you will probably have some tests to diagnose your particular bladder type. Although these are described below, it is important that you not depend on labels to describe your bladder.

Upper Motor Neuron Bladder (Reflex or Spastic Bladder)

The upper motor neuron (reflexic or spastic) bladder tends to hold smaller volumes of urine than before an injury. Just like your other muscles, your bladder muscles may have spasms and contract on their own. The result is that you may have frequent, small urinations with varying amounts of voluntary control, depending on the severity of your neurologic injury. This activity is common in SCI above the sacral level.

Lower Motor Neuron Bladder (Flaccid Bladder)

In the lower motor neuron (flaccid or are-flexic) bladder, the bladder muscle has lost its ability to contract and can be easily stretched,

allowing large volumes of urine to accumulate in the bladder. Because the muscle does not contract, urine may leak from the bladder when it is over-distended (overfilled). The urine "spills over" like a glass that is too full of water. This bladder activity is common when SCI affects the sacral cord—cauda equina, the spinal nerves below the sacral cord.

In both types of bladders, sensation of fullness is impaired.

BLADDER FUNCTION TESTS

There are a number of tests that can evaluate the structure and function of the urinary system. Because they are all commonly done, the tests are described here to prepare you in advance. You may have one or several of them.

Imaging Procedures

KUB (Kidneys, Ureters, Bladder)

Plain x-ray visualizes the abdomen and surveys the urinary tract.

Ultrasound

In the ultrasound, sound waves (like sonar) are bounced off tissue surfaces, and an electronic picture is produced on a screen. Variations in the image can detail the structures or anatomy and thus define problems.

This test is useful in identifying tumors, cysts, and stones in the urinary tract. It also is used to measure the prostate, testicles, and other organs in the abdomen.

Renal Scan

The purpose of a *renal (REE-null)* scan is to assess the function and the blood supply of the kidneys. It is done by injecting a radioactive substance into a vein and then "reading" counts over the kidneys. The amount of radioactivity is extremely low.

Intravenous Pyelogram (IVP)

An IVP is an x-ray study in which an intravenous injection of contrast material containing *iodine* is given. The contrast is excreted by the kidneys and shows up on x-ray. A series of films is taken to show the size, shape, and working order of the kidneys, ureters, and bladder. It can also show the size and number of kidney stones, if present.

PLEASE NOTE that if you have ever had an allergic reaction to IVP dye, be sure to tell your physician.

Your bowel needs to be empty for this test, so do a good bowel program the evening before or the morning of the test. You may also have to refrain from eating and drinking the night before the test. The nursing staff will let you know if other preparation is necessary.

Cystogram

In this test, contrast material is injected into the bladder via a catheter. This test shows the size and shape of the bladder, as well as if urine moves backward through the system from the bladder up to the kidneys (reflux). This condition is due to excess pressure in the bladder, and is one cause of kidney damage, which needs to be detected and treated early.

Bladder Filling Studies

Cystometrogram

A *cystometrogram (siss-toh-METT-roh-gram)* (CMG) shows how your bladder reacts when it is filled with either carbon dioxide (CO2) or water. This mimics the way it would usually react when filled with urine. A urethral catheter is inserted for this test. The test measures the amount of pressure that builds in your bladder. With this information your practitioner can help plan a bladder program best suited for you.

Urodynamics

Urodynamics (yurr-oh-die-NAMM-icks) is a broad term that refers to a series of diagnostic techniques used to evaluate the bladder. Tests that may be part of this urodynamics evaluation include a cystometrogram, measurement of urethral pressures, as well as EMG (electromyograph) of the external sphincter.

This comprehensive study will assist in planning the best bladder management program for you. If there are changes in your bladder function over time, you may need this study repeated.

Cystoscopy

Cystoscopy (siss-TOSS-koh-pee) involves the urologist looking at the inside of your urethra and bladder through a lighted, hollow, specialized telescope inserted through the urethra. This is used in diagnosing and sometimes treating problems occurring inside the bladder.

Other Laboratory Tests

There are a number of tests evaluating the blood and urine that show how your urinary system is functioning:

Creatinine (kree-AT-en-een) clearance

This test involves collecting all of your urine for a 24-hour period. It is an important indicator of kidney function.

Urine cultures

A urine specimen is sent to the laboratory to look for bacteria. When a sensitivity test is also ordered, specific antibiotics that kill these bacteria can be determined.

Urinalysis

Urine is analyzed for a number of different chemical and cellular products.

Blood ureanotrogen (BUN) and creatinine: This blood test monitors renal function.

BLADDER MANAGEMENT

There are a number of basic goals in bladder management:

- Have *low bladder volumes*
- Have *low bladder pressures*
- Avoid infections
- Keep your skin dry

Bladder volumes are kept low by:

- Watching your fluid intake
- Routinely emptying your bladder

If you have an incomplete injury, you may with time regain some or all voluntary control of your bladder.

If you have a complete injury, one or a combination of the following bladder emptying techniques will become part of your bladder management program.

Bladder Emptying Techniques

Intermittent Catheterization

A small rubber or plastic tube is inserted into the bladder to drain urine several times a day. We refer to the process as an *intermittent catheterization program*, or ICP. The nursing staff generally does ICP initially. As you become more involved in your care, you or your attendant will be taught so you can continue this at home.

If you are managing your bladder with ICP, you will be asked to keep your bladder volume around 300 to 500 ml/cath. Adjust the frequency and the interval of catheterizations and the fluid intake to produce a minimum of 1,500 cc/day of urine output. You should catheterize at least four times per day and, depending on your fluid intake, you may catheterize more often.

Important note: More than 500 cc in your bladder overstretches your bladder muscle and makes you prone to infection or reflux. (See the section in this chapter on "Avoiding Infections.")

Indwelling Catheter

Two types of continuous drainage are *urethral (foley)* and *suprapubic catheters*. A foley catheter is a hollow tube with a balloon on the end so when inflated it will stay in your bladder. This is placed through your urethra (urine channel) and is usually changed one time per month. A suprapubic catheter is placed in your bladder through a small opening in your lower abdomen. This is a surgical procedure. Once the opening is made you or your attendant can change the catheter about once a month, just like a foley. This catheter also has a balloon to keep it in your bladder.

Stimulated Voiding

Some bladders can be mechanically stimulated to empty. Just as a spastic muscle may move when tapped or brushed, so may a UMN bladder. "Reflex voiding" may be induced by tapping over the lower abdomen or tugging on pubic hairs.

Spontaneous Voiding

Some UMN bladder muscles spontaneously contract. For those who have bladders that trigger on their own or who have had a *sphincterotomy (SFINK-turr-AH-tom-ee*, surgery to open the bladder "gate"), wearing an external collecting device or *condom catheter* will keep you dry. There are many different types of condoms, and your SCI team will work with you to find the best device for you.

Keeping Bladder Pressures Low

High bladder pressures before the bladder empties can cause urine to "back up" (reflux) into the kidneys, causing damage. Two such conditions are:

1. *Irritable bladder*—loss of bladder compliance, meaning the bladder has lost its elasticity, so that high pressures are generated with increasing volumes of urine. It is not advisable to use valsalva or crede maneuvers to empty the bladder with known high pressures.

2. *Dyssynergia (DISS-inn-URR-jah)*— the bladder contracts but the sphincter will not open. It is like trying to press the air out of a mattress with the plug closed. Autonomic dysreflexia can also occur with dyssynergia. (See the chapter on "Autonomic Dysreflexia.") To keep pressures low, keep your volumes low and treat the dyssynergia. Dyssynergia can be treated by either the use of medication to relax the sphincter or by surgery to open it up.

Avoiding Infections

1. Maintain a consistent fluid intake to "wash out" bacteria and to limit stone formation.

2. Empty your bladder routinely and prevent overdistension. More than 500 cc can weaken your bladder muscle in two ways. First, the muscle cells cannot fight off infection as well. Second, the muscle cannot contract as tightly and leaves behind a pool of urine in which bacteria can grow.

3. Sterile catheterization is performed while you are in the hospital. You will be taught a "clean" technique for home management before discharge. In some instances you may do a clean catheterization while in the hospital.

4. If you are taking any medication related to your bladder management, make sure you follow the practitioner's recommendations.

Keeping Your Skin Dry

The best way to keep your skin dry is to carefully follow your bladder management program.

1. Routinely empty your bladder by the method that works best for you.

2. Manage your fluid intake.

3. Wear appropriate appliances. These include condoms/external devices or padding specific to you.

4. Avoid infections. Infections may make your bladder irritable, which can cause frequent incontinence between intermittent catheterization or leakage around foley or suprapubic catheters.

5. Change your clothes as soon as they are wet.

PROBLEM SOLVING

People with SCI are at risk for infection because mechanical methods are needed to empty the bladder. Infections are caused by bacterial growth. Three sites of infection common to SCI are the kidney, bladder, and testicles.

A kidney infection is called *pyelonephritis (PIE-ell-low-neff-RIGHT-iss)*; a bladder infection is called *cystitis (siss-TIE-tiss)*; and an infection involving the testicles is called *epididymitis (epp-eh-DID-ee-MIGHT-uss)*.

Table 6.A will help you understand these infections and the diagnostic tests and treatments that may be required.

Kidney Damage and Kidney Failure

Kidney failure is a complex combination of conditions. Basically, it means that your kidneys do not function properly. Infections, stones, or reflux can damage your kidneys.

TABLE 6.A. Types of Infection

TYPE OF INFECTION	SIGNS AND SYMPTOMS*	DIAGNOSTIC TESTS	TREATMENT	OTHER CONSIDERATIONS
Kidney (pyelonephritis)	• Chills • Fever • Flank pain • Hematuria (bloody urine) • Urinary frequency • Cloudy, thick urine • Foul smelling urine • Sediment • Burning upon urination • Increased spasticity • Autonomic dysreflexia	• Urinalysis • Culture + sensitivity (C+S)	• Increased fluid intake • Antibiotics • Foley catheter possible	Re-evaluation of bladder management
Bladder (cystitis)	Same, although you may not have a fever & chills	• Urinalysis • Culture + sensitivity (C+S)	• Increased fluid intake • Antibiotics • Usually not necessary to insert foley	Chronic attacks require re-evaluation of bladder management
Testicles (epididymitis)	Any of the above, plus: • Hot, red swollen scrotum • Testicular pain in incomplete lesions	• Urinalysis • Culture + sensitivity (C+S) Plus: • Scrotal ultrasound	• Increased fluid intake • Antibiotics • Foley possible • Bed rest • Scrotal support to elevate scrotum • Hot & cold compresses to scrotum	Re-evaluation of bladder management

*You may not have all of the signs and symptoms.

Your kidney function will be addressed during routine annual check ups.

Autonomic Dysreflexia

If your SCI is at the sixth thoracic level (T6) or above, you may develop autonomic dysreflexia. It is important that you read the chapter on "Autonomic Dysreflexia." You will need to know the symptoms and how to take care of this condition immediately, as this can be a serious problem!

Urinary Stones

Stones can develop in the kidneys, ureters, or bladder. They are collections of mineral deposits, which can develop because of infection, high-calcium levels, or an increase of other chemicals in the blood and urine. They usually are small enough to pass through the urinary system and appear in the urine as sediment that looks like sand. If they are large, they may block the urinary system and could damage your kidneys.

Table 6.B will help you understand urinary stones. Stones may develop without your realizing it, so your yearly evaluation will evaluate your system. Sometimes you may have the symptoms outlined in table 6.B.

TABLE 6.B. Urinary Stones

SIGNS AND SYMPTOMS	DIAGNOSTIC TESTS	TREATMENT	OTHER CONSIDERATIONS
(You may not have all of them.) • Excruciating pain in lower back or lower abdomen, which may radiate to groin (for those who have sensation) • Nausea • Vomiting • Anxiety because you may not know why you are uncomfortable • Frequent infections • Fever and chills • Bloody urine	• Blood specimen • Urinalysis • IVP • Cystocopy	Care is individualized depending on stone, but may include: • Increased fluids • Straining urine • Taking medication • Having surgery	Re-evaluation of bladder management

Important: **If at any time you see blood in your urine, call your doctor or the SCI clinic.**

WHAT IS THE BOWEL?

The *bowel*, also called the *colon*, is the *large intestine*, the last part of your digestive system. The waste products of digested food are stored in it until you need to have a bowel movement.

HOW THE DIGESTIVE SYSTEM AFFECTS BOWEL MOVEMENT

Your diet, the amount of exercise you do, and the regularity of your bowel movements play an important role in keeping you healthy. The following is a description of the digestive system and how some parts can affect your bowel movements. *(See figure 7.1.)*

- *Mouth*: As you chew, saliva mixes with broken-up pieces of food. If you eat a well-balanced diet high in fiber, there will be enough bulk to make passage through the system run smoothly.

- *Esophagus (eh-SOFF-ah-guss)*: This is a hollow passageway through which food reaches the stomach.

- *Stomach:* Digestive juices break down the food into carbohydrates, fats, proteins, and other end products. (See the chapter on "Nutrition" to find out why these things are important.)

- *Small intestine*: As the watery mixture moves through here, nutrients are absorbed into the blood stream.

- *Bowel (large intestine) or colon*: Water is absorbed back into the body as the remaining by-products of digestion move through the bowel. When these by-products move through the bowel too

quickly, your bowel movements are very watery. This is called *diarrhea*. When these by-products remain in the bowel for prolonged periods of time, water continues to be absorbed into the body. This results in hard and difficult to pass stools. *Constipation* is the medical term for this. SCI may affect the last half of the large intestine causing slow, uncoordinated passage of stool.

- *Rectum:* When stool reaches the rectum, you get the urge to have a bowel movement. If you have a lack of feeling in your rectum, you will not get this urge.

- *Anus*: This circular muscle is the sphincter (gate) of your rectum. When you relax this

FIGURE 7.1. The Digestive System

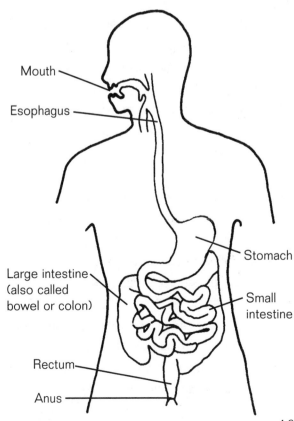

Mouth

Esophagus

Stomach

Large intestine (also called bowel or colon)

Small intestine

Rectum

Anus

muscle, you can have a bowel movement. When you tighten it, you can prevent having a bowel movement. If you are unable to relax or tighten this sphincter, your bowel movements cannot be controlled.

BOWEL PROGRAM

A bowel program is the total combination of diet, exercise, fluids, medication, and scheduled bowel care. The goals of your bowel program are to prevent bowel accidents (unplanned bowel movements), to produce bowel movements at regular and predictable times, and to minimize bowel-related complications.

Bowel Care

Bowel care is the scheduled process of starting and assisting your body to have a bowel movement. Bowel care is part of the bowel program. Bowel care is the procedure for assisting bowel movements that can be learned and followed in a series of steps.

Good control of your bowels after a spinal cord injury is possible with planned bowel care as part of a bowel program. Keeping your bowel emptied on a regularly scheduled basis to prevent chronic over-distention is the goal. Using an abdominal binder to support the abdomen may be helpful.

To stimulate peristalsis (wave-like movement of the intestines), you may use a rectal suppository, mini-enema, and/or digital stimulation of the rectal muscles. Scheduled bowel care can be done on a commode, on a toilet, or in bed with pads, whichever works best for you.

The types of things you will need included in your bowel care as part of your overall bowel management program will be best determined by the type of bowel you have

following your SCI, whether it is reflexic or areflexic. The rehabilitation nurse and your health-care provider will work with you to establish the most effective bowel care routine. The following is a description of things and techniques that are commonly used in bowel care regimes. Table 7.A lists some medications that may be prescribed as part of your bowel program.

Do:

1. Establish a regular time for bowel care that will fit into your daily schedule. Your actual bowel care can be every day, every other day, or every three days. In the first weeks after your spinal cord injury, your bowel care will be every day.

2. Eat a well-balanced diet with high-fiber foods.

3. Have privacy.

4. Be comfortable.

5. Exercise regularly (range-of-motion exercises).

6. Drink as much liquid as your bladder management will allow.

Don't:

1. Use large enemas, because they decrease normal bowel muscle tone. Mini-enemas may be prescribed.

2. Take strong oral laxatives routinely.

Supplies Needed

- Suppository inserter (if you need one)
- Suppository or mini-enema
- Lubricating jelly
- Waterproof pads
- Gloves
- Antibacterial soap and warm water
- Toilet paper or moist wipes for cleansing
- Scissors if using mini-enema

TABLE 7.A. Bowel Medications

TYPE OF MEDICATION	MEDICATIONS	WHAT IT DOES
ORAL LAXATIVES		
Stimulants	Bisacodyl, Cascara, Castor Oil, Senna	Increase the wave-like action of peristalsis to move stool through the bowel faster and keep it soft.
Osmotic Laxatives	Lactulose, Magnesium Citrate, Magnesium Hydroxide, Magnesium Sulfate, Sodium Biphosphate, Sodium Phosphate	Increase stool bulk by pulling water in the colon. You need to drink extra fluids with these.
Bulk-forming laxatives	Hydrophilic Muciloid, Methylcellulose, Psyllium	Add bulk to stool. You will need to drink extra fluids with these.
Stool softeners	Docusate Calcium (DOSS), Docusate Potassium, Docusate Sodium, Mineral Oil	Help stool retain fluid, stay soft, and slide through the colon.
Prokinetic agents	Metoclopramide	Stimulate bowel peristalsis.
RECTAL STIMULANTS		
Suppositories	Bisacodyl	Increases colon activity by stimulating the nerves in the lining of the rectum.
	CO_2	Produces carbon dioxide gas in the rectum, which inflates the colon and stimulates peristalsis.
	Glycerin	Stimulates peristalsis in the colon and lubricates the rectum to help pass stool.
Enemas	Mineral oil	Lubricates the intestine.
	Mini-enema	Stimulates the rectal lining and softens stool.

Table 7.A was adapted from *Neurogenic Bowel: What You Should Know*; Consortium for Spinal Cord Medicine Clinical Practice Guidelines; page 27, March 1999.

HOW TO PERFORM BOWEL CARE

If you have sufficient upper extremity function, you will learn to do your own bowel care. If you are not able to do your own bowel care, you will learn to instruct others in the process.

Do your bowel care about 30 to 45 minutes after a meal or hot drink, because this stimulates peristalsis to promote stool movement in your colon. If you use intermittent catheterization procedure (ICP) to empty your bladder, you should do it before bowel care.

1. *Washing Hands:* Wash your hands and put on a clean pair of exam gloves. Hand washing is important to maintain a clean environment and decrease the risk of infection that can be caused by stool contamination.

2. *Set Up and Positioning:* Arrange all the supplies you will need so they are easily within reach when you are ready for them. Many people sit up on a commode chair for bowel care, as gravity may help with emptying the bowel. Some transfer to the commode chair after medication insertion (step 4) while others position themselves on the commode chair first. Others do their care in bed for a variety of reasons. If you are side lying in bed, the left-side-down position is usually recommended.

3. *Checking for Stool:* Put on an exam glove and lubricate a finger. Check rectum for stool and gently remove any stool that may be there. Be sure to use a water soluble lubricant.

4. *Insertion of Stimulant Medication:* If you need stimulant medication, insert a well-lubricated suppository high up into your rectum with a gloved finger or adaptive

device. Place it right next to the intestinal wall *(see figure 7.2)* to allow the medication to come in contact with all surfaces of the rectal wall to provide optimal stimulation. Another medication choice may be an enema. An enema tip should be gently inserted into the rectum to the neck of the container. Squeeze the container and wait 5-15 seconds before removing the tip.

5. *Waiting Period:* Wait 5-15 minutes after insertion of any stimulant medication.

6. *Digital Stimulation:* Digital stimulation is a technique that can both start and enhance the strength and frequency of peristalsis. Do digital stimulation by gently inserting a lubricated gloved finger or adaptive device into your rectum. With a firm circular motion, rotate your finger maintaining contact with the bowel lining all the way around until it relaxes (15-60 seconds). You may need to do digital stimulation every 5-10 minutes to promote and prolong peristalsis while the anus relaxes.

FIGURE 7.2. Suppository Placement

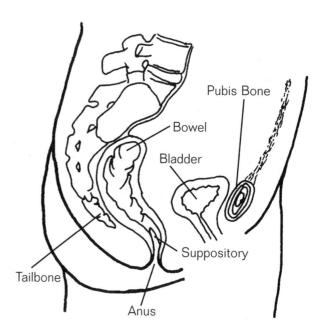

This allows stool to pass through the anus until gas and stool flow have stopped.

7. *End of Bowel Care:* Do a final check with lubricated glove or adaptive device to determine if rectum is empty. Other signs that bowel care may be complete are: if no more stool has come down after 2 digital stimulations or if mucus is coming out without stool.

8. *Clean Up:* Wash and dry the anal area and your hands.

Autonomic Dysreflexia

If you experience symptoms of autonomic dysreflexia (AD) during bowel care, you may need to use an anesthetic cream (contact your health-care provider for prescription) for medication insertion and digital stimulation. Please refer to the chapter on autonomic dysreflexia for further information.

Things That Can Affect Your Bowel Program

1. Exercise stimulates peristalsis. Range of motion can be done before bowel care or after inserting the suppository and before digital stimulation. Your routine use of your wheelchair, even an electric wheelchair, is also exercise.

2. Some medications can affect peristalsis. For example, many narcotics or anticholinergics may slow down peristalsis and cause constipation.

3. Emotional stress may cause either constipation or diarrhea.

4. Change in time of scheduled bowel care may lead to bowel accidents.

5. Your diet can harden or soften your stool. *(See table 7.B.)*

TABLE 7.B. Dietary Effects on Bowel Management

FOOD GROUP	FOODS THAT HARDEN STOOLS	FOODS THAT SOFTEN STOOLS
Milk	Milk, yogurt made without fruit, cheese, cottage cheese, ice cream	Yogurt with seeds or fruit
Bread & Cereal	Enriched white bread or rolls, saltine crackers, refined cereals, pancakes, waffles, bagels, biscuits, white rice, enriched noodles	Whole grain breads and cereals
Fruits & Vegetables	Strained fruit juice, apple sauce, potatoes without the skins	All vegetables except potatoes without the skin
Meat	Any meat, fish, or poultry	Nuts, dried beans, peas, seeds, lentils, chunky peanut butter
Soups	Any creamed or broth-based without vegetables, beans, or lentils	Soups with vegetables, beans, or lentils
Fats	None	Any
Desserts & Sweets	Any without seeds or fruits	Any made with cracked wheat, seeds, or fruit

PROBLEM SOLVING

Diarrhea

Diarrhea is frequent loose or watery stools, which may cause unplanned bowel movements and accidents.

Causes

1. Spicy foods or foods containing caffeine: coffee, tea, cocoa, or many soft drinks

2. Medications such as antibiotics; or an increase or decrease in medications you are already taking

3. Over-use of laxatives or stool softeners

4. Severe constipation

5. Flu or intestinal infection

6. Psychological stress

Solutions

1. Eat the recommended foods for when you have diarrhea *(see table 7.B)*.

2. Stop any laxatives until diarrhea clears up.

3. Stop stool softeners temporarily, then begin after diarrhea is over, adjusting dose to get the stool consistency you want.

4. Evaluate whether there is a chance that you have an impaction or blockage: no stools, hard stools, or small, hard bowel movements within the last week. One of the most common causes of diarrhea is an impaction where only liquid and soft stool can get past the impaction. Call your SCI clinic or physician.

5. After diarrhea clears up, re-evaluate your bowel program, use of stool softeners, diet, etc.

6. Try eating yogurt with active cultures when taking antibiotics to help restore the normal bacterial flora in your bowel.

7. Call your health-care provider if diarrhea lasts more than 24 hours.

Constipation

Constipation is a common condition in which stool does not pass as often, as fast, or as completely as we usually expect. The stool may be hard and dry. It is sometimes hard to determine if you are constipated until you have had incomplete results or no results after 2 or more episodes of bowel care. Be sure you know the amount of stool produced with each bowel movement.

Causes

1. Lack of a regularly scheduled bowel care

2. Incomplete emptying during bowel care

3. Diet low in fiber

4. Bed rest or low physical activity levels

5. Medications: Narcotics, iron, aluminum hydroxide, or an increase or decrease in medications you are already taking

6. Dehydration

Solutions

1. Do bowel care on a scheduled basis. You may need to increase the frequency of bowel care.

2. Eat foods high in fiber to help prevent constipation; see the chapter on "Nutrition."

3. Increase activity, range of motion.

4. Take psyllium hydro-mucilloid (Metamucil).

5. Take docusate sodium (DOSS).

6. Drink plenty of fluids as tolerated by your bladder program.

7. Try milk of magnesia or senna the night before scheduled bowel care.

8. Talk to your health-care provider about trying a rectal stimulant medication, or a stronger one if you are already using one, for your bowel care.

Impaction

An impaction is a partial or complete blockage in the intestine by stool.

Causes

Same as for constipation.

Solutions

1. Manually remove stool in rectum.
2. Call your health-care provider for advice.

Rectal Bleeding

Rectal bleeding is seen as bright red blood on your stool, toilet paper, or glove.

Causes

1. Hemorrhoids
2. Hard stools (constipation).
3. Rectal fissures (cracks or breaks in the skin).
4. Traumatic digital stimulation of anus (for example, long fingernails damaging the rectum during digital stimulation).
5. Bleeding from higher up in the gastrointestinal tract.

Solutions

1. Soften stools with DOSS, psyllium powder, or increased fluid intake.
2. Do gentle digital stimulation using much lubrication.
3. If bleeding continues for two to three bowel care episodes, consult your health-care provider.
4. If bleeding does not stop between scheduled bowel care episodes, consult your health-care provider immediately.

Autonomic Dysreflexia

See the chapter on "Autonomic Dysreflexia."

Causes

Anything that can cause pain, such as:

1. Hemorrhoids or fissures
2. Full or overdistended bowel (constipation, skipped bowel care, impaction)
3. Rough digital stimulation

Solutions

1. Regularly scheduled bowel care with adequate emptying. You may have to increase the frequency of the scheduled bowel care you do.
2. Comfortable positioning during bowel care.
3. Anesthetic ointment applied to anal area 5-10 minutes before suppository insertion and digital stimulation.

No Bowel Movements for Two to Three Scheduled Bowel Care Episodes

Causes

1. Constipation
2. Impaction
3. Not eating

Solutions

1. Try to determine cause.
2. Call your health-care provider.

Excessive Gas

Causes

1. Gas forming foods (*see table 7.C*)
2. Constipation
3. Swallowing air while eating or drinking
4. More than normal bacterial breakdown of bowel contents

TABLE 7.C. Foods that may Cause Gas

VEGETABLES

Beans (kidney, lima, or navy)
Broccoli
Brussels sprouts
Cabbage
Cauliflower
Corn
Cucumbers
Kohlrabi
Leeks
Lentils
Onions
Peas (split or black-eyed)
Peppers
Pimentos
Radishes
Rutabagas
Sauerkraut
Scallions
Shallots
Soybeans
Turnips

FRUITS

Apples (raw)
Avocados
Cantaloupe
Honeydew melon
Watermelon

Solutions

1. Eat your food slowly, chewing with your mouth closed; avoid gulping food.

2. Certain foods may give you gas. Do trial periods of omitting these foods one at a time to enable you to determine which, if any, cause you to have excess gas.

3. Begin a scheduled bowel care regime.

RESOURCES

Publications

Neurogenic Bowel: What You Should Know: A Guide for People with Spinal Cord Injury

Purchase:

PVA Distribution Center
P.O. Box 753
Waldorf, MD 20604-0753
(888) 860-7244
www.pva.org.

Bowel Management Programs: A Manual of Ideas and Techniques

Purchase:

Accent Press
Accent Special Publications
Cheever Publishing, Inc.
P.O. Box 700
Bloomington, IL 61702
(309) 378-2961

Taking Care of Your Bowels

Purchase:

VA San Diego Healthcare System
Spinal Cord Injury Unit
3350 La Jolla Village Dr.
San Diego, CA 92161
(800) 331-8387; (858) 552-8585
(858) 552-7541 TTY

Taking Care of Your Bowels—The Basics

Taking care of Your Bowels—Ensuring Success

Purchase:

    Northwest Regional Spinal Cord Injury
      System
    University of Washington
    Department of Rehab Medicine
    1959 NE Pacific
    Seattle, WA 98195
    (800) 366-5643; (206) 543-3600

Download: depts.washington.edu/rehab/sci

Home Care Manual for Spinal Cord Injury

Purchase:

    Santa Clara Valley Medical Center
    751 S. Bascom
    San Jose, CA 95128
    (408) 885-5000

Preventing Secondary Medical Complications: A Guide for Personal Assistants to People with Spinal Cord Injury

Purchase:

    Research Services
    UAB, Department of Physical Medicine
      and Rehabilitation
    619 19th Street South, Room 529
    Birmingham, AL 35249-7330
    (205) 934-3334

Download: www.spinalcord.uab.edu

Fact Sheet #10: *Bowel Management in Spinal Cord Injury*

Purchase:

    Arkansas Spinal Cord Commission
    1501 North University, Suite 470
    Little Rock, AR 72207
    (800) 459-1517

Download: www.state.ar.us/ascc/Publications/
publications.html#factsheets

Videos

SCI Video Access, a lending program
  of information videos
Spinal Cord Injury Network International
3911 Princeton Drive
Santa Rosa, CA 95405-7013
(800) 548-2673; (707) 577-8796
www.spinalcordinjury.org/videos.htm

What should you eat to stay healthy? Hardly a day goes by without someone trying to answer that question. Newspapers, magazines, books, radio, and television give us a lot of advice about what we should or should not eat. Unfortunately, much of this advice is confusing.

Some of this confusion exists because we do not know enough about nutrition to identify an "ideal diet" for each individual. People differ, and their food needs vary depending upon age, sex, body size, physical activity, and other conditions such as a spinal cord injury. Some guidelines for "healthy" people are listed below.

- Eat a variety of foods.
- Maintain ideal weight.
- Avoid too much fat, saturated fat, and cholesterol.
- Eat foods with adequate starch and fiber.
- Avoid too many sweets.
- Avoid too much sodium.
- If you drink alcoholic beverages, do so in moderation.

EAT A VARIETY OF FOODS

You need about 40 different nutrients to stay healthy. These include vitamins, minerals, protein, carbohydrates, fats, and water. These nutrients are in the food you eat.

No single food item supplies all the essential nutrients that your body needs. Therefore, you should eat a variety of foods to ensure an adequate diet.

One way to ensure variety and a well-balanced diet is to select foods each day as suggested by the food guide pyramid. *(See figure 8.1.)*

FIGURE 8.1. The Food Guide Pyramid

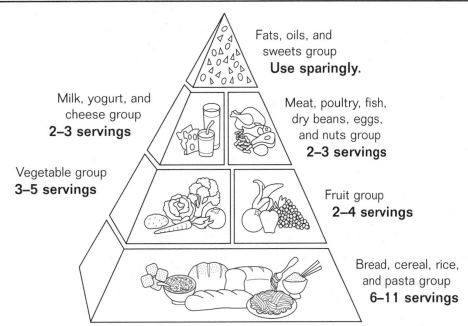

Fats, oils, and sweets group
Use sparingly.

Milk, yogurt, and cheese group
2–3 servings

Meat, poultry, fish, dry beans, eggs, and nuts group
2–3 servings

Vegetable group
3–5 servings

Fruit group
2–4 servings

Bread, cereal, rice, and pasta group
6–11 servings

If you eat a wide variety of foods, you will not need to take a vitamin or mineral supplement. However, if you are not able to eat the recommended number of servings from each level of the food guide pyramid, a multi-vitamin and mineral supplement may help you meet your nutritional needs; check with your doctor or dietitian first.

MAINTAINING AN IDEAL WEIGHT

If you are too heavy, your chances of developing some chronic disorders are greatly increased. Obesity is associated with diabetes, high blood pressure, and increased levels of blood fats. This can lead to *atherosclerosis* (*ath-urr-oh-sklurr-OH-siss*) or hardening of the arteries. These can increase your risk of having heart attacks or strokes. Obesity also increases your risk of developing pressure sores, impairs mobility, and makes transfer difficult.

If you are underweight, you may have a decreased ability to fight infections and may tire more easily. You may also be at risk for development of pressure sores. Being underweight is also associated with a shortened lifespan.

Therefore, try to maintain your "ideal" weight. But how do you determine what is an ideal weight for you? There is no absolute answer for this, but table 8.A lists acceptable weight ranges for most people with SCI. Ask your doctor or dietitian what your ideal weight is after your spinal cord injury.

Weight Loss

Do you need to lose weight? If so, you must take in fewer calories than you burn. This means that you must either select foods containing fewer calories, or you must increase your activity, or both. Listed below are some ways to help you lose weight.

- Limit the size of your food portions.
- Avoid second servings.
- Eat slowly, allowing at least 20 minutes per meal.
- Enjoy every bite.
- Make eating a separate activity.

TABLE 8.A. Acceptable Weight Ranges

HEIGHT (feet/inches)	WEIGHT (pounds)
MEN	
5'1"	123–129
5'2"	125–131
5'3"	127–133
5'4"	129–135
5'5"	131–137
5'6"	133–140
5'7"	135–143
5'8"	137–146
5'9"	139–149
5'10"	141–152
5'11"	144–155
6'0"	147–159
6'1"	150–163
6'2"	153–167
6'3"	157–171
WOMEN	
4'9"	97–106
4'10"	98–108
4'11"	99–110
5'0"	101–113
5'1"	103–116
5'2"	106–119
5'3"	109–122
5'4"	112–125
5'5"	115–128
5'6"	118–131
5'7"	121–134
5'8"	124–137
5'9"	127–140
5'10"	130–143
5'11"	133–146

- Try not to skip breakfast or lunch and try to avoid overeating at dinner.
- Avoid using food as a way of dealing with boredom, anger, fatigue, or anxiety.
- Consciously choose food with a view to its nutritive value.
- Avoid keeping high-calorie, low-nutrient snacks around the house.
- Eat less fat and fatty foods.
- Eat less sugar and sweets.
- Eat only when you are hungry.
- Be active.
- Know the danger period during the day when you tend to overeat. Be prepared with other alternatives.
- Be forgiving. No one is perfect. If you fall off your diet one meal or day, compensate by eating less the next meal or day.

Lose weight *gradually* to allow your body to adjust to the change. One to two pound weight loss per week is safe. If you lose weight gradually, you are less likely to regain the weight when you reach your goal. Long-term success depends upon the development of new and better habits of eating and exercise. If you desire to lose weight, your dietitian can help you plan a diet that meets your individual needs.

Weight Gain

If you need to gain weight, do so gradually. A steady gain of one to two pounds per week will allow your body to increase in muscle mass and not just fat. Listed below are some ways to help you gain weight.

- Consume at least three balanced meals per day.
- If you have a decreased appetite, eat six small meals per day.

- Eat foods that have higher fat content, such as whole milk, milkshake, or eggnog; raw vegetables with dip; cream soups.
- Add extra margarine, peanut butter, jelly, or jam to bread and crackers.
- Use thick gravies and cream sauces.
- Eat high-calorie snacks between meals, such as dried fruit, nuts, ice cream, and milkshakes. If you are busy during the day, carry your snacks with you.
- Make mealtime as pleasurable and relaxed as possible by planning your meals ahead of time and eating with a friend. Avoid arguments during mealtime.
- Prepare foods that look good and are tasty.
- Eat foods that fill you up quickly at the end of the meal. For example, liquids and high-fiber foods (salads, vegetables, fruits).

AVOID FAT AND CHOLESTEROL

Both saturated fat and cholesterol are known to increase your risk of developing heart disease.

- *Saturated fats* are fats that harden at room temperature, such as butter. They are found in animal products and in coconut, palm, and other vegetable oils that have been converted to a saturated fat through a process called *hydrogenation (high-DRAHJ-in-AY-shun).*
- *Cholesterol* is a wax-like substance found in every cell of the body. It is an essential component of cell membranes. It is found in food that comes from animal sources. However, it is not required in our diet because our liver makes all we need.

How to Avoid Too Much Fat, Saturated Fat, and Cholesterol

- Choose lean meat, fish, poultry, dry beans, and peas as your protein sources.
- Moderate your use of eggs (to three per week or less) and organ meats (such as liver).
- Limit your intake of butter, cream, hydrogenated margarine (solid margarine), shortenings, coconut oil, and foods made with these products.
- Trim excess fat and skin off meats.
- Broil, bake, or grill rather than fry food.
- Read labels carefully to determine both amounts and types of fat contained in foods.

NOTE: Do not avoid fats if you are underweight. Focus on monounsaturated and polyunsaturated fats.

EAT FOODS WITH COMPLEX CARBOHYDRATES AND FIBER

The primary sources of energy in the average U.S. diet are carbohydrates and fats. If you limit your fat intake, you should increase your daily amount of complex carbohydrates to supply your body's energy needs.

In trying to reduce your weight to "ideal" levels, carbohydrates have an advantage: they contain less than half the number of calories per ounce than fats.

Complex carbohydrate foods are better for you than simple carbohydrates. Simple carbohydrates such as table sugar, syrup, and honey provide calories but little else in the way of nutrients. Complex carbohydrates such as beans, peas, nuts, seeds, fruits, vegetables, whole grain breads, and cereals contain fiber and many essential nutrients in addition to calories.

The average American diet is relatively low in fiber. *Fiber* (roughage, bulk) is a strand-like material. It cannot be digested by the human stomach because it resists digestive enzymes. Therefore, fiber helps with your bowel program and keeping you regular. Regularity can be a problem for people with a spinal cord injury.

To make sure you get enough fiber and complex carbohydrates in your diet, you should eat fruits and vegetables, whole-grain breads, and cereals. Examples of foods that are high in fiber are listed below:

Breads and Cereals

- All bran cereals, some cereals with whole wheat or raisins, whole wheat bread or whole rye bread, cracked wheat bread. Read the labels on cereal boxes.
- Brown or unpolished rice.
- Potatoes, baked or boiled in their skin.
- Cracked wheat, barley, and millet.

Fruits

- Fresh oranges, apples, pears, all types of berries, grapes, peaches, plums.
- Dried fruits, such as raisins, prunes, peaches, apricots, dates, figs.

Vegetables

- Cabbage, celery, chicory, cucumbers, escarole, lettuce, tomatoes, carrots.
- Cooked vegetables, such as all types of beans, greens (beet, mustard, collard), broccoli, kale, squash, brussels sprouts, corn.

Legumes, Nuts, and Seeds

- Soybeans, kidney beans, lima beans, split peas, walnuts, peanuts, sunflower seeds, pumpkin seeds.

AVOID TOO MANY SWEETS

The major health hazard from eating too many sweets is *tooth decay*, but other concerns are that sweets are *high in calories* and *low in the amount of nutrients* that your body needs. Therefore, if you need to lose weight, limit the amount of sweets in your diet.

If you do not need to lose weight, sweets may be added to your diet after you have consumed the amount of servings recommended in the food guide pyramid.

How to Avoid Excessive Sugars and Sweets

- Use less of all sugars, including white sugar, brown sugar, raw sugar, honey, and syrups.

- Eat less of foods containing these sugars, such as candy, soft drinks, cakes, and cookies.

- Select fresh fruit or fruits canned without sugar or with light syrup rather than heavy syrup.

- Read food labels for clues on sugar content. If the words sucrose, glucose, maltose, dextrose, lactose, fructose, or syrups appear first, then there is a large amount of sugar.

- Remember, how often you eat sugar is as important as how much sugar you eat.

AVOID TOO MUCH SODIUM

Table salt contains sodium and chloride; both are essential elements. Too much sodium, however, is a hazard for people who have high blood pressure or heart disease. It also can cause *edema (swelling due to water retention)*.

Sodium is present in many beverages and foods that we eat, especially in certain processed foods, condiments, sauces, pickled foods, salty snacks, and sandwich meats. Baking soda, baking powder, monosodium glutamate (MSG), soft drinks, and even many medications (many antacids, for instance) contain sodium. Therefore, it is not surprising that adults in the United States take in much more sodium than they need. Since most Americans eat more sodium than is needed, consider reducing your sodium intake. Use less table salt. Eat sparingly foods to which large amounts of sodium have been added. Remember that up to half of your sodium intake may be "hidden," either as part of the naturally occurring food or, more often, as part of a preservative or flavoring agent that has been added.

How to Avoid Too Much Sodium

- Learn to enjoy the unsalted flavors of foods.

- Cook with only small amounts of added salt.

- Add little or no salt to food at the table.

- Limit your intake of salty foods, such as potato chips, pretzels, salted nuts and popcorn, condiments (soy sauce, steak sauce, garlic salt), cheese, pickled foods, cured meats.

- Read food labels carefully to determine which foods have sodium in them.

TABLE 8.B. Alternative Seasonings to Use Instead of Salt

SPICES	USES
All spice	Ground meats, stews, tomatoes, peaches
Basil	Eggs, fish, lamb, ground meats, liver, stews, salads, soups, sauces, fish cocktails
Bay leaves	Meats, stews, poultry, soups, tomatoes
Caraway seeds	Meats, stews, soups, salads, breads, cabbage, asparagus, noodles
Chives	Salads, eggs, sauces, soups, meat dishes, vegetables
Cider vinegar	Salads, vegetables, sauces
Curry powder	Meats, chicken, fish, tomatoes, tomato soup
Dill	Fish sauces, soups, tomatoes, salads, macaroni
Garlic (not garlic salt)	Meats, soups, salads, vegetables, tomatoes
Lemon juice	Meats, fish, poultry, salads, vegetables
Marjoram (sweet)	Soups, sauces, salads, lamb, pot roast, pork, veal, fish, vegetables
Mustard (dry)	Ground meats, salads, sauces
Onion (not onion salt)	Meats, vegetables, salads
Paprika	Meats, fish, stews, sauces, soups, vegetables
Parsley	Meats, fish, soups, salads, sauces, vegetables
Rosemary	Chicken, veal, meatloaf, beef, pork, sauces, stuffings, potatoes, peas, lima beans
Sage	Meats, stews, biscuits, tomatoes, green beans
Savory	Salads, egg dishes, pork, ground meats, soups, squash, green beans, tomatoes, peas
Thyme	Eggs, meats, sauces, soups, peas, onions, tomatoes, salads
Tumeric	Meats, eggs, fish, sauces, rice
Wine	May be used in marinades

• Use herbs and spices to season your food. Go lightly—a little goes a long way. Enhance the food flavor, don't overwhelm it! Start with a quarter teaspoon per four servings. Some common spices and their uses are listed in Table 8.B.

DRINK ALCOHOL IN MODERATION ONLY

Alcoholic beverages tend to be high in calories and low in other nutrients. Even moderate drinkers may need to drink less if they wish to achieve ideal weight.

On the other hand, heavy drinkers may lose their appetites for foods containing essential nutrients. Vitamin and mineral deficiencies occur commonly in heavy drinkers—in part because of poor intake, but also because alcohol alters the absorption and use of some essential nutrients.

Heavy drinking may also cause a variety of serious conditions, such as *cirrhosis (sir-ROW-sis)* of the liver and some neurological disorders. Cancer of the throat and neck is much more common in people who drink and smoke than in people who do not. If you drink, you should do so in moderation.

Moderation

- One or two 6-ounce glasses of wine.
- One or two 12-ounce bottles of beer.
- One or two 1-ounce shots of 80-proof hard liquor.

RESOURCES

Web Sites

www.eatright.org

This website is maintained by the American Dietetic Association (ADA), the world's largest organization of food and nutrition professionals. The site includes food and nutrition news, a marketplace, nutrition resources, "find a dietitian," and other information. The ADA promotes nutrition, health, and well-being. It publishes the *Journal of the American Dietetic Association*, a monthly journal on food and nutrition topics for professionals and consumers. Its programs include government affairs, which monitors food and nutrition-related regulations and legislation; education and registration for nutrition professionals; information on insurance coverage for nutrition services; and a

nutrition hotline. The hotline, at (800) 366-1655, provides recorded messages on nutrition topics and referrals to dietitians.

American Dietetic Association
120 S. Riverside Plaza, Suite 2000
Chicago, IL 60606-6995
(800) 877-1600

www.mayohealth.org

This is Mayo Clinic's Health Oasis, maintained by the Mayo Foundation for Medical Education and Research. Health Oasis provides information about patient care, research, and education programs. The website's Nutrition button offers news, a reference library, recipes, a searchable cookbook, food quizzes, and more.

Mayo Clinic
200 First Street, SW
Rochester, MN 55905
(507) 284-2511
(507) 284-9786 TDD

navigator.tufts.edu

Tufts University Nutrition Navigator, a Rating Guide to Nutrition Websites, is maintained by the Center on Nutrition Communication of Tuft's School of Nutrition Science and Policy. As a response to the proliferation of websites offering nutrition advice, the Tufts advisory panel reviews and rates websites for their content (accuracy, depth of information, frequency of updates) and usability. Sites can receive a ranking up to 25; sites that rank below a certain level on accuracy will not be listed. The ADA site received a rating of 23; the Mayo Clinic site 25.

The purpose of this chapter is to teach you about medications in general. This is not like most material written about medications. Other pamphlets and books tell you the details of specific types of medication. This chapter focuses on the things you should know about medicine. This includes how they work, why they come in varied forms, and how to read medicine advertisements. But more than that, it centers on what it means to be a smart consumer. All of this will help you to work with your doctor and health-care team to better plan your medications.

Each person is unique and may require different dosages or have varied responses to certain medications. Side effects will not always occur in every person who takes a given drug. Ask your medical staff to recommend what is best for you.

HONESTY IS THE BEST POLICY

The biggest part of the help you give is honesty. You will need to give your doctor a complete medical history and a list of your current medications, both prescription and over-the-counter. This should include any "natural" alternative supplements. Your medical history tells your doctor what kinds of reactions, illnesses, and problems you have had. These are very important in understanding your past treatment and planning your future care.

You must keep in mind that medications not only affect your body, but they also affect other medications as well. For example, even if you are taking something as simple as

aspirin, it may defeat the ability of some other drug to work. (For more on this, see the section in this chapter on drug interactions.) Certain over-the-counter drugs like cold remedies can affect your bladder and bowel medications.

PREGNANCY

If you are pregnant or suspect that you may be, tell your doctor. Any time that you are taking medication, your baby is taking it too. Depending upon the type of medication, it can have serious results.

HOW DRUGS DO WHAT THEY DO

The starting point of how drugs work is knowing that your body is mostly made of chemicals. Medicines are chemicals too. When you take drugs, they mix with the chemicals of your body.

Drugs work in two ways. One kind of drug works just the way it is, in the same form it was when you took it. Others work only after your body has broken them down into some other form so that they can mix with the chemicals and tissues in your body.

Most drugs are not things your body would normally use, so you eventually get rid of them through urine, bowel movements, tears, sweat, or your lungs. Each drug takes a certain amount of time to go through your body. This affects the dosage you are given. For example, some drugs pass very quickly through your body. Others are meant to build up and have a lasting effect.

Drugs Come in Different Forms

The drugs you take come in many different forms. There are tablets, capsules, syrups, chewables, injections, or ointments, to name a few. The form the drug comes in depends on how it is supposed to work in your body. Below are some examples of drug forms and how they are used.

- *Chewable tablets:* Fast-acting, often given to children.

- *Swallowed tablets, capsules:* Long-acting. They must be swallowed whole so that all the medicine is not released at once, but over time.

- *Injections*: For fast-acting effects or for drugs that cannot be taken orally and digested (such as insulin).

- *Syrups*: Mostly cough medicines, they are usually thick, and may contain sugar.

- *Suppository/enema*: Medicines that are taken through the rectum. For those who cannot swallow medicine, medications that may cause nausea, or some medications that act directly on the rectum.

- *Ointment/creams/lotions*: Mostly for skin conditions. An exception is nitroglycerin gel, sometimes used to treat autonomic dysreflexia.

- *Suspensions*: Contain large amounts of solid medication suspended in liquid. The solid tends to settle to the bottom, so you must be sure to shake the bottle before using in order to mix the contents.

- *Skin/transdermal patches:* Release medication slowly into your body by absorption through your skin. Be sure to apply the patch to a clean, dry skin area that has little or no hair and is free of scars or irritation. Remove the previous patch before applying a new one. Do not try to trim the adhesive patch to adjust the dosage.

- *Inhalers:* Contain medicine that must be inhaled to work properly. It is best to receive instructions on how to correctly use the inhaler delivery system, and ask a health-care professional to watch you give yourself a dose. Read directions carefully, because some inhalers require rinsing your mouth out with water afterwards.

- *Eye drops:* Should be applied only after you wash your hands. Do not let the tip of the applicator actually touch the surface of your eye.

Side Effects

It is important to know about possible side effects from medications before you take them. Your pharmacist, doctor, nurse, or other member of your health-care team should explain this to you. It is also important to tell your doctor about any side effects that concern you after you take the medication. It is a good idea for you to learn both the generic and brand names of your medicines. Make a list of all the medicines you take, and keep this with you at all times. This is important when you need routine or emergency medical care.

Side effects are classified in various ways:

- *Pharmacologic (FARM-ah-co-LODGE-ick) effects:* These are the chemical side effects of the drug itself. They are often predictable and controllable. In addition, many drugs do more than one thing in your body. The size of the dosage you are taking can make a big difference. In some cases, your body may just need time to adjust to the drug or its side effects.

- *Allergic reactions:* Allergic reactions come in many forms, showing up immediately or even as late as several weeks after the medication is taken. Skin reactions are the most common symptom. They range from redness and itching to swelling and sores. Allergic reactions have nothing to do with the action of the drug or the size of the dosage. They are often unpredictable in occurrence, except that people who have allergies such as hay fever tend to react more to medications. Reactions of this kind are a good reason why your medical history needs to be complete. There may be less of a chance that a reaction will occur if your doctor knows about your past experiences with medications.

If you do experience some kind of reaction to your medication, call your doctor immediately. You may need to stop using it.

- *Anaphylaxis (ANN-ah-fill-AX-iss):* A severe, immediate response to a drug. It is a life-threatening situation of decreased blood pressure and difficulty breathing. Stop using it immediately and CALL 911.

- Drug interactions: This refers to the effect two or more drugs have on each other. Sometimes, one drug helps another work. Other times, one stops the other. Occasionally, both keep on working, but their actions combined create yet another action.

Alcohol is likely the drug most often combined with other drugs. For example, alcohol more than doubles the effect of tranquilizers. Keep in mind that cough syrups contain enough alcohol to have the same effect. Alcohol should not be taken with any medications.

Again, the best policy is to tell your doctor about any drug you take on a regular basis. Even if it's just aspirin, it could make a big difference.

Over-the-Counter, Prescription Drugs, and Herbal "Natural" Preparations

The foremost difference between the over-the-counter medications and prescription medications is that medicines sold over the counter have a wider margin of safety. This means that they have fewer and milder side effects and little or no chance of addiction. Herbal ("natural") preparations include diet supplements, botanical phytomedicines, vitamins, minerals, and other substances. See the chapter on "Alternative Medicine" for more information.

This does not mean that over-the-counter medications or natural supplements are harmless. Used unwisely or along with other drugs you are taking, they can affect your health a great deal. So tell your doctor if you are using any over-the-counter medicines, natural supplements, or any prescription medications.

Many herbal supplements are added now to various food items. Be sure to read the label, and be careful about eating something that would interact with your medications. See the chapter on "Alternative Medicine" for more information.

WHAT DOES YOUR PRESCRIPTION SAY?

Most prescriptions include the following elements

1. Your name and address.
2. "Rx"-the symbol marking the area where the actual prescription is written.
   - The name and strength of the drug.
   - The quantity to be prepared.
   - The directions of how to take the drug. (These are abbreviated on the prescription but will be written out for you on the drug container.)

3. Refill information.

4. The date.

5. The prescriber's name, address, and registration number.

6. The prescriber's signature.

In most cases, your doctor will be able to give a drug order to the pharmacy over the phone. However, this cannot be done with prescriptions for controlled substances. These include such drugs as narcotics and stimulants. They can only be obtained with a written prescription taken to the pharmacy. Refills for your prescriptions are convenient to get with refill order forms. *(See figure 9.1.)* Be sure to send in refill orders to your pharmacist in plenty of time, at least two weeks, to ensure you do not run out of medication.

Refill forms contain almost the same information as your original prescription, except that this one keeps a running tab on how many refills you have used and are still allowed. As long as you still have refills on your original prescription, you will get an updated refill order form for your next refill. If you have used your last refill, you will get a form for reordering the whole prescription. This form only works with your doctor's signature. Most pharmacies, clinics, and hospitals use a computerized system to facilitate ordering your medications and keep track of refills.

Refill laws limit the number of refills you can have written onto a prescription. Drugs are put into different categories that tell how many refills they may have.

ADVERTISEMENTS ABOUT MEDICINES

As a consumer, you should be aware of *all* the information about a drug, not just what the advertising source says. Check with your doctor about what you should take. Do not be fooled by advertising. Read it carefully, and if you still have questions, ask your doctor or pharmacist.

FIGURE 9.1. Sample Prescription Refill Form

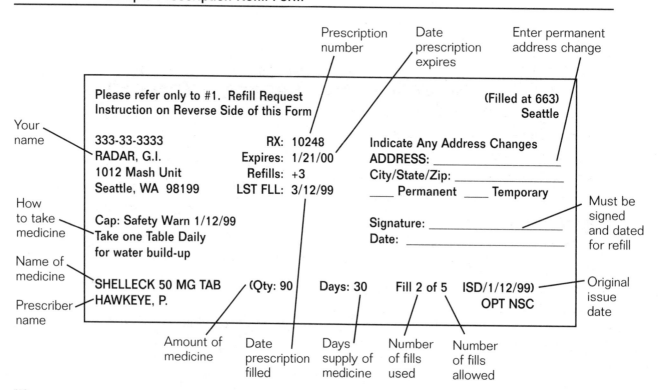

AT HOME

In the hospital, you have many people around you to make sure that you take your medications safely. They tell you how much to take and when to take it. They will also tell you about what you are taking and how it works.

At home, you will be the only one responsible for your medicine chest. You are responsible for taking your medication on time and in the proper dosage. Be aware of any changes that may occur while you are taking your medication and let your doctor know about them.

Being responsible also means that you have to keep yourself informed about what you are taking. *Read the labels of everything you take.* If you still have questions, ask your pharmacist. This applies to both your prescription and over-the-counter medications.

The information you read about medications does not make you an expert in planning your own medication. Planning drug therapy is a science. Consumer guidelines cannot replace the medical knowledge that your health-care team has. Your pharmacist can assist you in understanding your medications and how to take them safely and effectively.

RESOURCES

Publications

Advice for the Patient: Drug Information in Lay Language, Volume II, 19th edition

Purchase:

The United States Pharmacopeial
Convention, Inc.
Micromedex, Inc.
6200 S. Syracuse Way, Suite 300
Englewood, CO 80111

The Pill Book: *The Illustrated Guide to the Most-Prescribed Drugs in the U.S.* H. Silverman. CMD Publishing. Bantam Books, 1997.

The Johns Hopkins Complete Home Encyclopedia of Drugs. S. Margolis. Medletter Associates, Inc. 1999.

The Medical Advisor: The Complete Guide to Alternative and Conventional Treatment. Time-Life Books, Alexandria, Virginia. 1996.

Web Sites

www.mayohealth.org
The Mayo Clinic's Health Oasis website has an icon for Medicine. It leads you to news, a searchable drug guide, "Ask the Physician," reference articles, links to other sites, and more.

www.healthtouch.com
Healthtouch Online allows you to search for information on specific drugs. Information provided includes generic and brand names, dosages, side effects, and more. Individual drug companies are credited with information on specific drug pages.

www.virtualdrugstore.com
This site provides basic information use, side effects, and cautions on prescription and nonprescription drugs.

Nerves, Muscles, and Bones |

Chapter 10

A number of different conditions can affect your nerves, muscles, and bones after spinal cord injury. The sections in this chapter will describe each situation, its advantages and disadvantages, and what you can do about it.

SPASTICITY

When some spinal cord nerve cells are disconnected from your brain, they gradually develop exaggerated activity due to increased reflexes. Even simple things like touching or irritation to your skin, stretching muscles, or stretching your bladder may cause a reflex contraction of your muscles that you cannot control. One common type of reflex muscle contraction seen after spinal cord injury is a rigid straightening of the knees and pointing of the toes *(extensor spasms)*. Another type is bending of the hip and of the knee *(flexor spasms)*.

Advantages of Spasticity

* Increases in spasticity can warn you of any pain or problem in those areas where you cannot feel (e.g., urinary tract infection, pressure sore).
* Spasticity helps maintain your muscle size and bone strength.
* Spasticity helps promote circulation of your blood.
* You may learn to use your spasticity functionally; for example, using extensor spasms to help transfer or to walk with braces.

Disadvantages of Spasticity

* It may interfere with sleep, driving, sex, walking with braces, etc.
* It may cause scraping of your skin and result in skin breakdown.
* It may cause limited joint movement. See the section in this chapter on contractures.

What to Do

Most spasticity can be tolerated to enable you to benefit from its advantages. Some ways to control spasticity and prevent complications include:

* Performing daily range-of-motion exercises to help reduce spasticity.
* Avoiding stimulation that you find aggravates the spasticity (such as fast movements or certain body positions).
* Asking your therapists about the use of padded straps and splints that can help control spasticity.
* Protecting your feet and legs from striking sharp or hard objects due to a spasm (such as against your wheelchair during transfers).
* Taking a warm (not hot!!) bath or shower.
* Trying to relax or reduce your level of stress.

If spasticity is interfering with sleep, driving, or other functioning, you should discuss treatment options with your SCI physician. Treatment alternatives include:

* Medications, although all have side effects and none will eliminate spasticity.

- Injections of specific medications into muscle or nerve to reduce spasticity.
- Surgery to nerve roots or the spinal cord.
- Baclofen pump—surgical implantation of a device that delivers medication directly to the spinal canal.

Remember that significant increases in spasticity may be a sign that something is wrong in a part of your body where you do not have sensation. Such increases in spasticity might be a warning of a urinary tract infection, a pressure sore, a kidney stone, appendicitis, an ingrown toenail, or almost any problem. Notify your SCI physician, nurse, or therapist if you notice a significant increase or decrease in spasticity.

ATROPHY AND CONTRACTURES

Atrophy is the shrinking of muscle size when the muscle is not used. Some spinal cord injuries result in more, some in less, atrophy. A *contracture (con-TRACK-churr)* is the tightness of tissues around joints and in muscle that limits movements and function.

Contractures can be a serious problem, but they are preventable. If range-of-motion exercises are neglected, then contractures can permanently limit joint movements. Contractures can interfere with transfers or daily activities. They can also change your posture, which can lead to pressure sores. In some individuals, tightness of some muscles of the hand is actually planned to improve the grip, called *tenodesis (ten-oh-DEE-siss)*.

Atrophy generally is not a medical problem.

Treatment

Contractures can be prevented by moving joints through their full range of motion regularly. Joints in body areas where the muscles do not work must be moved manually by yourself or by an attendant. Your therapists will instruct you in the range-of-motion exercises most important for you and how they should be performed. Shoulders, elbows, hips, knees, and ankles are the joints that usually are most important in preventing contractures. If you have severe spasticity, then range-of-motion exercises may be particularly important, and you may need to do them several times a day.

Atrophy is generally not treated directly. Instead, you will learn to avoid any long-term pressure on bony areas (such as buttocks or shoulders) to prevent pressure sores. Atrophy can sometimes be prevented by electrical stimulation performed two or three times per day. However, *each* muscle that is to be increased in size must be stimulated, and this can become very time consuming and costly. Unless some functional movement returns or unless this electrical stimulation is medically necessary, this strengthening is not generally done with SCI patients.

NEUROGENIC HETEROTOPIC OSSIFICATION

Neurogenic heterotopic ossification (nurr-oh-JENN-ick HETT-air-oh-TOP-ick OSS-ih-fih-KAY-shun), or NHO, is the growth of a knot-like piece of bone in the soft tissues of your body below the level of your spinal cord injury. This bone is formed in between your muscles, often near a joint. It can affect all joint areas below the level of your spinal cord injury. It most commonly affects

FIGURE 10.1. Neurogenic Heterotopic Ossification

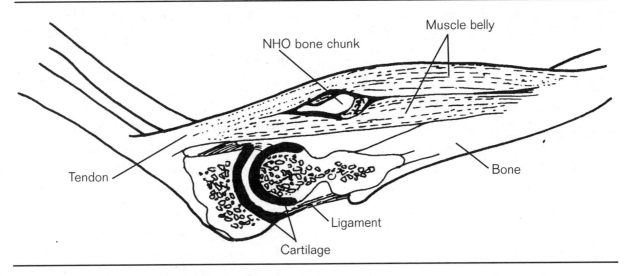

the areas of your hips, knees, and elbows. *(See figure 10.1.)*

Ultimately the bone growth stops on its own. It usually will appear on an X-ray about 4 to 10 weeks after the process begins. The whole process ends in about 8 to 30 months, leaving behind a chunk of complete, honest-to-goodness bone. It is just like any other bone in your body except that it serves no particular function, and it can often cause problems in joint movement.

The Cause

Unfortunately, the cause of this condition is unknown. *It does not occur in all people with SCI.* No one knows why some patients get it and others do not. For some reason, your bone cells show up in soft tissue, where they mature and harden.

Some things that may contribute to and start this process are probably related to changes in your body due to your injury. It may have something to do specifically with changes in blood flow, hormones, or the chemistry in the area where the NHO starts. Some people feel that overly vigorous range-

of-motion exercises can tear the tissues and cause the problem. Other theories are that local bleeding in the area caused by an injury or tearing leads to the deposits of bone cells.

Symptoms

- Decreased joint range of motion— this may develop slowly or quickly
- Swelling
- Redness
- Increased skin temperature over this swollen region

Other Causes of These Symptoms

These other conditions can have the same types of symptoms and must be evaluated:

- An infection in the area
- A broken bone
- Bleeding into the muscle
- Deep vein *thrombosis (throm-BO-siss) (DVT)*

Your doctor may do different tests to find out which condition is actually causing the symptoms. DVT must be ruled out by your doctor *immediately*, as this is a life-threatening situation and must be treated promptly. See the chapter on "Circulation."

Effects

The worst complications of NHO are severely decreased range of motion and contractures. These greatly interfere with your self-care and mobility and could cause problems with sitting, lower extremity dressing, transfers, bathing, and walking.

Testing for NHO

Three tests are used to evaluate and follow neurogenic heterotopic ossification:

1. *Alkaline phosphatase (AL-kah-line FOSS-fah-taze)*: The level of alkaline phosphatase in your blood stays high throughout the period of active bone formation. It eventually drops back to normal values when the NHO stops growing.

2. *X-rays:* X-rays are used to confirm the location of the NHO and to estimate how mature the new bone is. An X-ray cannot tell how long it has been there.

3. *Bone scan:* A bone scan is the best test for diagnosing NHO. It can detect NHO about four weeks before an X-ray can.

Treatment

There is no one, successful treatment of NHO. A medication called *etidronate disodium (or Didronel®, DID-row-nall)* is sometimes prescribed to try to prevent the NHO from starting or continuing.

Your doctor will know that the NHO has fully matured when your alkaline phosphatase returns to normal again and a bone scan shows no more actively growing bone. The bone may then be removed surgically to improve your joint movement. If the bone does not cause you any movement problems, your doctor may decide to just leave it there.

Help through Range of Motion

We feel that full, gentle *passive or active assisted range-of-motion* exercises help rather than hurt. You should try to maintain the range that you have.

OSTEOPOROSIS OR WEAK BONES

Osteoporosis (OS-tea-oh-poor-OH-siss) is loss of calcium and phosphorus from bone. It is common following spinal cord injury. Bones that usually are kept strong through muscle activity and walking can no longer get what they need. Osteoporosis weakens the bone and makes it easier to break and slower to heal.

Osteoporosis in People with SCI

There are no proven treatments for reversing or preventing osteoporosis, although some experimental treatments are being tested. The primary treatment is to prevent fractures. So extra precaution should be used to prevent falls or striking your leg against an object during transfers. Follow the range-of-motion guidelines from your therapists to avoid putting excessive stress or pressure on bones. Walking with braces may help to limit the amount of osteoporosis that develops in the legs.

PROTECTING YOUR UPPER EXTREMITIES

Your upper extremities—your shoulder, elbows, wrists, and hands—are important. Using a wheelchair, especially a manual wheelchair, requires more work with your arms than they were used to when you walked. Over-use injuries can occur but are less likely if you follow some simple advice:

- *Cuts, Blisters, and Abrasions on Your Hands:* Wheelchair-push gloves can be worn to protect your hands. They are not essential if you have paraplegia, but if you cannot feel all or part of your hands, protective gloves are a good idea.

- *Carpal Tunnel Syndrome*: This is an inflammation of the tendons leading into the hand that can cause pressure on the nerve entering the hand, which will result in a painful or numb hand. This is an over-use syndrome and prevention is the best cure—avoid repetitive motion of the wrist, especially flexion (bending your wrist down) or extension (bending your wrist up).

- *Ulnar Nerve Compression*: The ulnar nerve courses very close to the surface at the elbow. (This is your "funny bone"—not so funny when you bang it.) Avoid leaning on your wheelchair armrests or desktops. If you do this for balance, talk to your therapist about your wheelchair set-up for better trunk support.

- *Tennis Elbow (Lateral Epicondylitis)*: This is an inflammation of the extensor tendons of the wrist and fingers (the ones you use in straightening your fingers and raising your wrist). Avoid excessive repetitive motion.

- *Shoulders*: Primary issues at the shoulders are biceps tendinitis and impingement syndrome. Biceps tendinitis is caused by over-use of the muscle—often from overhead reaching activities. Impingement syndrome is more complex. Both problems relate to muscle imbalance, poor posture, and often poor habits in transfers.

Prevention

Shoulder protection programs should include anterior stretching of the anterior shoulder, posterior shoulder and rotator cuff strengthening, and avoidance of impingement patterns. Impingement pattern means weight bearing with the hand at or above the height of the shoulders. All transfers should be done with hands down—as low as possible—with a forward bent posture, allowing counterbalance with your head and upper body to decrease the weight bearing on your shoulders. Never use an overhead trapeze or overhead grab bar. Your wheelchair should be set-up up by your therapist to optimize your posture and push mechanics. See your physical therapist for simple exercises that should be part of your daily routine if you push a manual wheelchair and do independent transfers.

Pain is an early indicator. If you have pain in one of your joints or part of your shoulder or arm and you didn't do something obvious to cause it, you should contact a therapist familiar with spinal cord injury to help you troubleshoot and solve the problem. Early intervention is best.

Other Upper Extremity Issues

- *Edema:* Especially for people with high quadriplegia, swelling of the hands can be a problem. This makes your hands more vulnerable to skin breakdown. Elevation and compression are the best management, combined with daily range of motion. Consult your occupational therapist for more advice on management. Chronic edema can be a symptom of other problems. When elevation and compression fail to reduce the swelling, contact your doctor.

• *Shoulder Subluxation:* Again, this is an issue primarily for people with high quadriplegia without normal shoulder muscula-ture. The problem here is gravity: the weight of the arm pulls the shoulder out of the socket. The result can be pain. The best prevention and management is to support the arm, so do not allow your arm to dangle, and do not allow anyone to pull your weight with your arms.

• *Elbows:* Support your arm, not your body, through your elbows. Consult your therapist for proper positioning.

Above all else, *autonomic dysreflexia (ot-toe-NAWM-ick dis-re-FLEX-ee-ah)* is an *emergency situation*. Read this chapter carefully to learn about it before autonomic dysreflexia happens or if you think you have it.

Autonomic dysreflexia is a complication that can be seen in almost anyone with a *spinal cord injury* above *thoracic level seven*. It is important to be able to recognize autonomic dysreflexia and know what causes it and how to treat it, as it can be life threatening. Table 11.A describes the symptoms. Figure 11.1 shows what happens in your body during an attack of autonomic dysreflexia.

TABLE 11.A. Symptoms of Autonomic Dysreflexia*

High blood pressure

Severe pounding headache

Seeing spots in front of your eyes

Blurred vision

Slow heart rate

Goosebumps above level of SCI

Sweating above level of SCI

Flushing of skin above level of SCI

Nasal stuffiness

Important: **Uncontrolled high blood pressure is the dangerous part of autonomic dysreflexia, for it may be high enough to cause a stroke.**

*You may not have all of them.

CAUSES

Autonomic dysreflexia is generally brought on by something that would have signaled pain or discomfort in you before your injury. Some possible causes are listed below, with the most common ones first.

1. A full or distended bladder (frequently caused by a plugged or twisted catheter)
2. Stool impaction (severe constipation)
3. Infections (of the bladder, etc.)
4. Tests and procedures (cystoscopy, gynecological exam)
5. Pressure sores (decubiti)
6. Traumatic pain (severe cuts or broken bones)
7. Hot and cold temperatures
8. Sunburn
9. Tight clothes
10. Pressure on the testicles or penis
11. Severe menstrual cramps, labor (uterine contractions)
12. Stomach ulcers
13. Some drugs (digoxin, etc.)
14. Ejaculation

What to Do

1. *Sit up if you are lying down.* This will decrease your blood pressure.
2. *Find and remove the cause.* Autonomic dysreflexia usually will not go away until the cause of the problem has been corrected.
   - *Check for bladder problems first.* If you do not have a catheter in place, catheterize yourself. Empty your bladder

FIGURE 11.1. How Autonomic Dysflexia Happens

The Body's Response to Pain

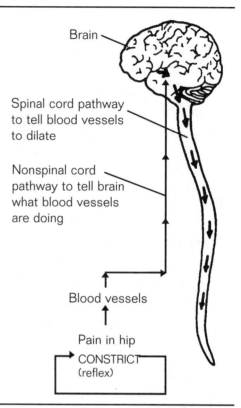

Before SCI

1. Blood vessels constrict by reflex activity and raise your blood pressure.

2. Nerves send messages up to the brain through your spinal cord, so you actually feel the pain.

3. Other nerves send messages up to the brain through automatic pathways other than the spinal cord to tell the brain what is happening to your blood vessels and blood pressure.

4. Brain then sends message down through the spinal cord to dilate (open up) your blood vessels, which will lower your blood pressure again.

After SCI

1. The same as before SCI.

2. You will most likely not feel the pain, because the messages cannot pass through the injured spinal cord.

3. The same as before SCI.

4. If your injury is at or above T7 level, your brain cannot get the dilation message back down to the blood vessels below your injury. The reason for this is that the area from T7 to T10 of the spinal cord sends messages to most of the blood vessels in your body. Your blood pressure stays high because the shut-off valve to lower your blood pressure does not work.

Important: **Autonomic dysreflexia is a vicious cycle that cannot be broken until you find the cause and remove it.**

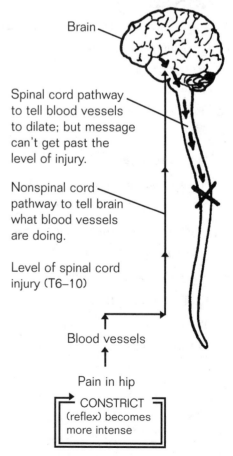

slowly by lifting the draining end of your catheter. If you empty your bladder too fast, you may cause it to go into spasm, which can cause your blood pressure to go up again.

- *Check for bowel problems next.*
  If your bladder is not the cause of the high blood pressure, check your bowel for stool. If there is stool in your rectum, you will need to remove it manually. Before removing the stool, you should apply numbing medicine, such as lidocaine, to the anus and then wait five minutes for the medicine to work. This will prevent further stimulation to the area, which can cause your blood pressure to go up even more.

- *Check for skin problems.* If neither your bowel nor your bladder seems to be the cause, strip yourself and look for cuts, bruises, or ulcers on your body.

3. *If the symptoms do not go away or your blood pressure continues to be high,* greater than 160 systolic, despite the above measures: apply nitroglycerin ointment to your skin above the level of injury or take hydralazine or nifedipine if your physician has given you this medication. This will lower your blood pressure while you are trying to find out why this has happened. Only certain patients who get autonomic dysreflexia a lot will be given this medication.

4. *GET HELP if you can't find the cause.* Call or go to the nearest hospital. Autonomic dysreflexia is an unusual problem, and not all health providers will know how to treat it. Present your Medical Alert Card for Autonomic Dysreflexia. (*See figure 11.2.*)

A physician should be notified immediately, because this is a medical emergency.

PREVENTION

You can prevent these symptoms in many cases, but not always.

Since the most common causes of autonomic dysreflexia are a full or distended (bloated) bladder and impactions of the bowel, you can prevent this from happening by making sure that:

- Your bladder is emptied routinely,
- Your catheter is draining well, and
- You have routine bowel movements.

You may be one of those people who just have this problem more often than others. In this case, your medical provider may put you on medication to prevent it. If you have problems with autonomic dysreflexia, you should have a blood pressure cuff at home and learn how to use it.

REMEMBER: If you do develop autonomic dysreflexia, you will soon learn what causes it for you. You will then be able to treat it quickly and effectively.

CARRY A CARD!

Figure 11.2 is an example of a card you can cut out and carry in your wallet. Put your name on the card in the space after "The bearer of this card." Let people know you have this card and use it with medical staff to instruct in emergency care. It may save your life!

RESOURCES

Publications

Autonomic Dysreflexia: What You Should Know

Purchase:

   PVA Distribution Center

   P.O. Box 753

   Waldorf, MD 20604-0753

   (888) 860-7244

www.pva.org

Available in Spanish.

FIGURE 11.2. Wallet Size Card for Autonomic Dysreflexia

Cut on Solid Lines   **Fold on Dotted Lines**

Medical Alert Card for Autonomic Dysreflexia

The bearer of this card,

_____,

is at risk for autonomic dysreflexia, a life-threatening complication of spinal cord injuries above the T7 level. It is caused by an exaggerated sympathetic nervous system response to a noxious stimulus below the level of injury. The usual etiologies of AD are inadequate emptying of the bladder, a full bowel, tight clothing, ingrown toenail, etc.

The symptoms can include elevated blood pressure, headache, nasal congestion, brady-cardia, and flushing (above the level of injury). Please note the normal blood pressure for an SCI patient is 90/60. If the AD is unresolved, it may result in myocardial infarction, stroke, retinal hemorrhage, or death. It is essential that the source be identified and the elevated BP be resolved immediately. Please see reverse of card for details of treatment.

Autonomic Dysreflexia Treatment

1. Raise the head of the bed up to 90 degrees or sit the person upright.
2. Check for the source of the AD: full bladder or bowel, tight clothing, ingrown toenail, pressure ulcer, or any other noxious stimulus. Removing the cause will usually eliminate or decrease the symptoms.
3. Monitor the blood pressure and pulse every 5 minutes.
4. Drain or irrigate the bladder, using a topical anesthetic jelly for catheterization.
5. Check the rectum for stool, after first applying an anesthetic ointment to the rectal wall. If stool is present, begin digital stimulation to promote reflex defecation.
6. If SBP is above 160, apply one inch of nitro paste to hairless skin, and cover with clear occlusive wrap.
7. If elevated SBP continues, apply one additional inch of nitro paste, to equal two inches.
8. Wipe off nitro paste when SBP decreases to 130
9. If SBP remains elevated despite two inches of nitro paste, give 10 mg of hydralazine. If SBP remains elevated after 10 minutes, give an additional 10 mg of hydralazine.
10. If SBP remains refractory to the above treatments, give 10 mg of bite-and-swallow nifedipine. If nifedipine is given, the patient is at risk for hypotension once the AD is controlled and must be monitored closely for several hours after administration of nifedipine.

Fold

A pressure sore or decubitus ulcer ("decube") is an injury to the skin and tissues below it. It is caused by excessive or prolonged pressure. When pressure is applied for too long, blood supply is cut off. This deprives the cells of oxygen and nutrients, which leads to skin breakdown.

The pressure on the tissues is always greatest right at the bone. Your tail bone (sacrum and coccyx), hips (trochanters), sit bones (ischials), or heels are the places to watch. Tissues here get squeezed between a "rock" (the bone) and a "hard place" (your chair or mattress, for example). Before your injury, your body signaled you to squirm around in a chair or change positions to get blood to an area. After spinal cord injury, you may not have the same warning system about your skin. Unless you think and then move by doing a "pressure release," the blood supply to an area can be cut off and result in a pressure sore.

Since pressure is greatest at the bone, the most damage is done there. A sore may look small at the skin's surface but can be much larger underneath. Think about this like the description of an iceberg: what you see on the skin (tip of the iceberg) is only a small part of the tissue damage underneath (the biggest part of the iceberg).

It is better to prevent a pressure sore. Even if you are able to heal a wound, especially a deeper wound, the skin and soft tissue below will never be as strong and elastic as before.

When you are at risk for pressure sores, the equipment you use should help relieve and distribute pressure over your bony areas. Special bed surfaces and wheelchair cushions can be chosen to help prevent pressure sores. But the most important prevention is to *MOVE YOUR BODY* frequently. If you do develop a pressure sore, *GET OFF IT. STAY OFF IT* until it is healed.

PRESSURE SORE CLASSIFICATION

A rating system is useful in identifying and describing the size and extent of a pressure sore. This is important so the treatment of your wound can be planned and carried out effectively. The deeper the pressure sore, the more serious the problem. The most common system for rating the severity of damage has 4 levels:

- *Stage 1.* This is an area of redness that does not fade or blanch. In darker skinned people, this may look dark red, blue, or purple. The skin is still intact.

- *Stage 2.* If the skin is broken open at all, the wound is at least a stage 2. This will look like a scrape, blister, or shallow crater.

- *Stage 3.* This wound will be a deeper crater, which goes all the way through the skin layer into the soft tissue below.

- *Stage 4.* This wound is deep enough to extend to a tendon, bone, or muscle.

COMPLICATIONS OF PRESSURE SORES

Sore Worsens

The length, width, and depth of a pressure sore can increase in size. In deep wounds, tunneling between layers of muscle, fat, or bone can occur. This is called *tracking*. Most of the time you can keep sores from getting worse by immediately getting off the sore and contacting your health-care provider. A pressure sore will not heal if pressure is still being applied to it.

Infections

Skin and wound infections can occur with pressure sores. In deep wounds, the bone can also become infected. This bone infection is called osteomyelitis. Sometimes this infection can spread into your bloodstream and make you very sick. By keeping your pressure sore clean and by following recommendations by your health-care providers, you can help prevent infections.

Scarring

The formation of scars is common as pressure sores heal. This scar tissue breaks down easier than normal skin without scars because scars have poor blood supply. Scar tissue is also less elastic and may not stretch enough as your body gets into different positions. Scarring of the skin and soft tissue may even decrease your range of motion in nearby joints.

Fortunately, scarring can be prevented by preventing deep pressure sores altogether. It is important not to let a superficial sore (which is likely to heal without a scar) turn into a deeper one. Even if deeper wounds heal, the area will have scar tissue.

HEALING SKIN BREAKDOWN

There are different ways to manage pressure sores after they have developed. Managing other body system problems that have an impact on wound healing is essential. Check with your health-care provider for the treatment plan that will work best for you. Some ulcers may even require surgical repair. All ways of treating pressure sores take a long time to work and require keeping pressure off the area (*see table 12.A*).

Pressure Management

The most important part of treating pressure sores is removing the cause. To treat any stage pressure area, remove pressure. For example, if the sore is on a pressure area related to sitting, don't sit until the problem is fixed. If your sore is on a pressure area related to lying down (like the tail or hip bones), don't lie in that position again until the problem is fixed. If this is a heel problem, eliminate pressure by wearing a special splint (for example a l'nard splint) or suspend your heel over the edge of a pillow.

Management of Other Body System Problems

Other problems can contribute to the development of a pressure sore. (*See table 12.B.*) For example, urine leakage that causes the skin to be wet for long periods of time can lead to skin breakdown. The urinary drainage must be managed in a different way. Another example might be spasticity that pulls you out of alignment in your chair causing uneven weight distribution and higher risk for skin breakdown. Your sitting posture must be corrected so you can have even weight distribution over your sit bones.

Anemia/Loss of Body Proteins

Healing skin requires good nutrition. If you are anemic or malnourished, healing will be slow. The pressure sore itself may cause anemia and malnutrition, especially if there is a large amount of drainage. Your health-care provider will give you advice about treating your anemia or low body proteins. You may need help from a dietitian to get enough of a well-balanced diet. You may need extra calories, protein, vitamins, and minerals.

Smoking impairs your skin's ability to heal due to constriction of blood vessels and limiting the absorption of some nutrients. If you have a pressure sore, try to stop using tobacco in any form. Call your health-care provider for help with stopping smoking.

Wound Care

If you develop a pressure sore, you should take immediate action. But before we talk about what to do if you have a pressure sore, you should know what *NOT TO DO*:

1. Don't massage areas of redness.

2. Don't clean your wound with soap, iodine (e.g., betadine), hydrogen peroxide, alcohol, vinegar, or bleach solutions. These solutions are toxic to your exposed tissues.

3. Don't try to dry your wound with a heat lamp or hair dryer.

4. Don't put sugar, vitamins, or antacids into your wound.

5. Don't use antibiotic ointments in your wound unless prescribed by your health-care provider.

If you have a MINOR skin breakdown, some simple wound care at home may allow healing to occur. Healing is promoted by keeping your wound moist (not wet) and covered. Rinse your wound with normal saline solution or by bathing in the shower. Blot the area dry, then cover with a film dressing (such as Tegaderm®) or a hydrocolloid dressing (such

TABLE 12.A. Time and Process for a Pressure Sore to Heal

STAGE	WHAT HAPPENS IN THIS STAGE	TIME SPAN
First Stage of Healing	The wound area gets red and hard to the touch. This happens because more blood and white cells are sent to this area to clear away dead tissue and to fight infection.	3–5 days
Second Stage of Healing	New blood vessels are formed to provide oxygen and nutrition to this area. This looks like bumpy, red tissue. At the same time, new cells are laid down at the bottom of the wound. After the first layer is formed, other cells grow underneath, filling in the wound. This is an *extremely* slow process. The sides of the wound are also building layers in the same way. The wound gets smaller, and scar tissue forms on the skin surface. In deep wounds, it is very important that the sides do not close in first. If they do, a pocket may remain in the middle of the wound and become infected. This space can become larger and may reopen the wound from the inside out.	1–21 days, depending on the size and depth of the wound. Can take much longer
Third Stage of Healing	Scar tissue becomes stronger and may fade in color, but scar tissue is never as strong as skin.	Up to 2 years

TABLE 12.B. Helping Pressure Sores Heal Faster

CONTRIBUTING FACTOR	ITS ROLE IN WOUND HEALING
Keeping weight or pressure off	This is the single most important thing you can do. Wounds will not heal if there is pressure on the area.
Oxygen	You need to have enough oxygen in your system for new cells to grow. You can help increase the amount of oxygen to your pressure sore by doing the following: 1. Range-of-motion exercises, but be careful not to rub the pressure sore on the bed 2. Stop smoking 3. Stay warm
Proper nutrition	Nutrition plays a key role in rapid wound helping. You can help by eating well-balanced meals, high in protein, three times a day. Adequate nutrition also helps to maintain your immune system, which helps fight off infection. Some valuable nutrients that help heal wounds are listed below. • *Carbohydrates:* Needed for energy source • *Proteins:* New cells are made from protein (tissue building) • *Vitamin C:* Needed to form and strengthen new blood vessels • *Vitamin A:* Needed to form new tissue cells and new blood vessels • *Iron:* Needed to form scar tissue • *Zinc:* Needed for healing to occur at its usual rate
Alcoholism	Frequently interferes with proper cell reproduction and is related to poor nutrition.
Stress	Raises blood pressure and muscle tension. With this, your body uses more energy, tires easily, and uses up the vitamins, minerals, and nutrients that are needed for healthy skin.
Diabetes	High-blood sugar slows the first stage of healing.
Anemia	Decreases the amount of oxygen to the healing tissue and slows reproduction.
Smoking	Causes blood vessels to narrow, reducing the amount of oxygen and nutrients getting to the wound.

as Duoderm®, Restore®, or Comfeel®). Your wound will make "soup" under these kinds of dressings. Don't be alarmed if there is a puddle of smelly drainage when you take off the old dressing—this is normal! If your ulcer does not heal or show progress toward healing within a week's time, call your health-care provider for guidance. A home care nurse may be needed to help manage your wound care.

If you have a deeper wound, or the wound has black, yellow, or gray tissue in it, or the skin around the wound has increasing redness, call your health-care provider right away.

SURGERY

Sometimes total pressure relief and good wound care are not enough to heal a pressure sore. In those cases, surgery may be needed. There are different surgical procedures depending on the location and severity of the pressure sore. Some procedures involve moving muscle and skin. Some also remove some bone. Each person with a pressure sore is evaluated for the procedure that will have the best chance of getting him or her back to living an active life.

There are limits to the number of times a pressure sore repair surgery can be performed. You are far better off preventing a serious sore.

Getting Ready for Surgery

Before surgery, the pressure sore needs to be well cleaned. This can take several weeks and may involve frequent dressing changes and/or surgically removing all the dead tissue from the wound.

If your sore is infected, your doctor may prescribe antibiotics. Signs of infection include redness and swelling around the wound, foul smelling drainage, and fever.

Also before surgery, your nutritional health will be evaluated to see if additional food (protein, vitamins, minerals) is needed to improve the chances of successful wound healing.

After Surgery

After surgery there will be a period of three to six weeks when you will stay in bed (usually a special bed) to allow the surgical site to heal. It is very important not to put pressure on the surgical site and not to pull or stretch the skin of that area. You will need help in turning. You will not be able to smoke for 3-6 weeks after your surgery. So plan to quit before hand.

After healing, range-of-motion exercises to the nearest joint will begin slowly. Next, there will be a gradual buildup of weight bearing or pressure on the site by lying or sitting on it in carefully planned sessions. This process of building pressure tolerance is very slow. Ask your nurse or doctor about this.

This surgical area will need special care for the rest of your life. It will never be as strong as it was before you had the pressure sore. Transfers and pressure tolerance will need to be regularly evaluated. Your seating system and how you do pressure releases may need re-evaluation.

The most important part of healing, whether by conservative methods or surgery, is for you to determine the cause of the pressure sore and to plan how it can be prevented in the future. For more general information about skin care, see chapter 2.

The first section of this chapter is primarily directed toward the newly injured individual. It discusses various reactions to disability and provides insights into adjustment. However, the "not-so-new" spinal cord injured person may enjoy reading this section too. You may find yourself reflecting on the early days after your own injury and re-examining the ways you relate to spinal cord injury. In addition, this section provides useful information about assertiveness training, stress management, relaxation training, time management, and setting priorities in your life. These are areas everyone can benefit from, whether they have spinal cord injuries or not.

Having a disability, such as a spinal cord injury, produces lots of questions about who you are; who you want to be; how other people, including your family, will interact with you; and how you live your life as a person with a disability. This chapter will offer some ideas and suggestions on ways to think about these personal questions. Unlike questions about your physical needs, personal and social questions have no exact answers or procedures to follow. What you decide to do with your personal and social life is up to you. Since some of these issues are difficult, this chapter will try to offer you some help.

In addition, this chapter includes information about independent living and your legal rights as a person with a disability. General self-improvement and civil rights books have made lot of nondisabled authors very rich, so you know these must be important topics! If questions regarding personal or family concerns come to mind, remember that you can talk to your social worker, psychologist, or other team member.

YOU ARE STILL THE SAME PERSON

Becoming spinal cord injured was probably the worst thing that has ever happened to *YOU*. *YOU* cannot change what has happened, leave it behind, or ignore it. One way or another, *YOU* have to deal with it. It's not easy.

To make a very important point, we've purposely emphasized the word *YOU* in the above paragraph. Many people each year are involved in accidents that result in spinal cord injury. Everyone is unique, and this does not change after injury.

YOU ARE STILL YOU!

There are many life experiences all rolled together that make you who you are and that is not going to change just because you may have to use a wheelchair now instead of legs for getting around. To put it another way, there is no reason to assume that your personality, intelligence, style of interacting with other people, and other personal traits will change as a result of injury. If you were smart, friendly, obnoxious, hard-to-get-along-with, finicky, argumentative, bossy, or goal-oriented before your injury, chances are very good that you will be the same way after injury.

Don't be surprised, however, if you experience intense sadness, frustration, and anger. These are normal human reactions that can occur in response to unfortunate things that happen to you. This is very common after injury and will lessen with time and new learning experiences. Tips on how to deal with these and other feelings and reactions are provided next.

EXAMINING YOUR FEELINGS TOWARD DISABILITIES

It's often said that one of the hardest things about coping with abrupt onset of disability is that you're suddenly thrust into it with all your able-bodied beliefs, attitudes, and misconceptions.

Do you know any people with disabilities? Are any friends or family members disabled? How about fellow employees or fellow students? If you have known someone well, you have probably discovered that the disability gradually seemed less important as the relationship grew. First impressions or initial attitudes are not always accurate, and they may change over time.

Many people have varying attitudes and impressions that show how they feel about people with disabilities. You may discover that you possess some of these beliefs as well, especially if your association with people with disabilities has been very limited or nonexistent. What are some common attitudes toward or first impressions about people with obvious physical disabilities? Here are some examples:

- Pity or sympathy for the individual, which often results in a condescending or patronizing attitude.

- Personal discomfort, anxiety, or fear of being around the individual with a disability. Therefore, such a person is actively avoided.

- Assumed cognitive/mental impairment because of physical disability.

- Assumed dependency because of physical disability.

- Assumed "second class citizen" status. People with disabilities may not be included in many activities or functions of their communities, or others may not treat them with equal respect.

- Unearned praise of the individuals because they are "so brave" or "have coped so well."

However, your attitudes about yourself and the attitudes of others (family, friends, and even strangers) can change. But beliefs do not change overnight. This is a gradual process that occurs with new learning and behaving. You may find that you are a "student" in the rehabilitation facility and a "teacher" on the outside who helps others to reassess their attitudes about physical disability.

THE ART OF LIVING

Each individual has a unique way of responding to major changes in lifestyle. How you respond to having a spinal cord injury is very personal and involves a wide variety of thoughts and feelings. Not everyone has the same experiences, but sometimes it helps to know that there are some problems that others have had to face. Others have found useful ways to cope with those problems, and these are available to you.

As mentioned earlier, it is important to consider "who you are." Some people prefer to ignore personal problems, others like to talk all the time, and others may want to call their favorite talk-show host or write to Dear Abby for advice. There are many ways to respond to personal needs and concerns. Most important, whether you read a book, talk with a friend, go to an educational group, or seek professional counseling, it is essential to choose what is best for *YOU.*

Almost all patients go through a "Why me?" phase when they are first injured. They ask themselves questions like, "Why did this happen to me?" "I always treated everyone fairly and did what I thought was right! So, why have I been singled out for this unfortunate thing to happen?" Or you may be saying, "I am being punished for all the wrongs I have done before my injury." Some patients bargain: "I promise to lead a good life from now on, if only I can be allowed to walk again." A very good book by Harold S. Kushner, *When Bad Things Happen to Good People*, describes these feelings in more depth.

Regardless of what conclusions you come to about why you were injured, you must reach some sort of conclusion and psychologically put the issue aside and look toward the future.

Different people accept change at different speeds. The process of accepting change is often called the "adjustment period." It is very difficult to estimate how long it will take you to adjust to your new lifestyle after being injured. What is important to you right after injury may not be as important later on in your life. The following example may help describe this process.

Imagine yourself learning to fly an airplane. Early on, you must learn a great deal of technical information and how to operate new, unfamiliar equipment. When you first sit in the cockpit, your attention is focused on the dials, levers, gadgets, and switches on the panels in front of you. After some basic training and practice, you will progress to the point at which you can fly to a given destination and not focus all your attention on gadgets or equipment. These things move to the back-

ground, and your attention is focused on the open sky beyond.

A similar process occurs after spinal cord injury. You first learn technical information about how your body works and how to operate new equipment like braces, wheelchairs, and catheters. After training and practice, you begin to focus your attention on other parts of your life.

The speed of your adjustment is greatly influenced by your philosophical attitude toward life. Some people's attitudes toward living are very flexible. They take each day as it comes. Others, though, are more rigid and have their lives planned for years to come. Their plans do not, of course, include a spinal injury. A good clue as to the progress of your adjustment is when you start thinking and verbalizing such statements as, "I wonder what the future holds for me" or "I would like to know what kind of work I could be trained to do with the amount of function I still have" or "What direction am I headed in now?"

Believe it or not, there is a positive side. Patients who have been injured for some years have said: "Life is richer for me now than it was before I became injured because I have slowed down. I have done much soul-searching in adjusting to my injury, and as a result, I have become a more mature and appreciative person. I am able to appreciate and admire things and qualities that in the past I would have missed." No one chooses to have a spinal cord injury, but as with most things in life, there is another side of the coin.

"NORMAL" FEELINGS

It is important to keep in mind that the personal and psychological issues you face will, over time, be less focused on your injury and have more to do with everyday life. The following discussion of feelings applies to emotions of crisis (right after your injury) as well as emotions that may come and go throughout your life. It is normal for people to experience a wide range of feelings after a major crisis. Anger, sadness, frustration, irritation, confusion, and isolation are common. How you feel is probably different from how others may feel. However, some people like to know that others have similar feelings. This section will discuss what you can do to help yourself in dealing with the emotional reactions you experience. Not all those emotions are going to be uncomfortable ones! The process of rehabilitation also involves humor, pride, hope, and a sense of accomplishment.

Anger

If you find yourself snapping at others, yelling when things go wrong or boiling over most of the time, know that many people experience anger. However, it may become difficult for you to work with others if that anger carries over into everything you do. A good test is to ask yourself: "Would I like to be treated the way I treat others?" If the answer is "No," ask yourself: "Who or what is getting in my way? Why am I angry?"

This kind of self-talk can help you step back from a problem, cool off, and develop a positive plan of action. Also, ask others to help you stay calm by talking about problems openly, rather than letting something build up to the boiling point and exploding in anger.

Humor

When was the last time you had a good, long, belly-shaking laugh? It seems that this type of "therapy" is often overlooked or discounted, especially when you are in the hospital. Recent medical writers have discussed the positive effect that laughing has upon both

mental and physical health. Norman Cousins, author of *Anatomy of an Illness as Perceived by the Patient*, discusses how he has used joke books, funny movies, and other forms of humor to help improve his ability to combat illness. Certainly, laughing is no "cure," but it can help you deal with difficult problems, and it usually sets up a positive mood.

Some suggestions to help you find humor are:

- Spend more time with friends who make you laugh.
- Go to a bookstore and look at joke books or humorous notecards.
- Read newspaper comics or comic books.
- Rent a video cassette recorder (with some friends) and watch a funny movie.
- Start a joke contest.

Sadness

It is very common for someone to feel intense sadness after a major loss or significant change in health. This is similar to the grief you might feel when someone close to you has died. Some people express this sadness with tears, withdrawal, avoidance of their usual routine, or talking about the sad feelings with a close friend. These are normal, common reactions. However, when these normal feelings seem to be overwhelming, persistent, or hopeless, you should consider getting help in dealing with your sadness.

The main differences between *grief* and significant *depression* are that depression is often accompanied by hopelessness, a sense of giving up, physical exhaustion, trouble sleeping, and a change in appetite. Try talking to someone close, thinking about something positive in your future, or maybe setting out to do something enjoyable (like listening to a concert, having a special dessert, or reading a good book). If you feel like "it's not worth trying," then talk with a member of your rehab team about those feelings. You can get some help.

Pride

How you feel about yourself is very important, especially in a rehabilitation setting. It influences how you look, talk, and act. Think of someone you know who is very proud and confident (not false pride). How do they look and act? When you feel good about yourself, other people will know because you care enough to groom well and present yourself nicely to others. This feeling starts when you tell yourself: "I am worthwhile as a person." Sure, you have faults, but you have some unique qualities as a person. You can learn to feel good about those qualities and that will begin to help you improve your sense of pride. A book called *A New Guide to Rational Living* by Albert Ellis and Robert Harper describes specific ways of improving and maintaining a positive sense of self-esteem and pride.

Frustration/Confusion

Having to try new ways of doing things can be both frustrating and confusing. First, try to identify the source of frustration. If you can identify a person, talk with that person about the problem as openly as you can. *Clear communication helps!* If talking about things makes you more upset, ask for a third party to help out or try to use some relaxation activities (mentioned later in this section) before you talk. *Being calm and relaxed can help!*

Sometimes you can identify why you are frustrated, but you can't figure out how to improve or change it. *Ask for help!* Another person can help you brainstorm, which may lead to a solution, or you may find a way to

stay relaxed in the face of some very frustrating situations.

LEARN TO LET OTHERS KNOW WHAT YOU NEED WITHOUT BEING RUDE

Many times, people feel upset, angry, and frustrated when they miss out on something they want. This section focuses on learning how to achieve certain things without hurting or stomping on others. This involves being assertive, without being nasty or aggressive.

There will be times when you need to ask for assistance with something you cannot accomplish on your own, or you may need to let someone else know they are doing something that really bothers you. Also, recent research has shown that people with spinal cord injuries often need to take the extra step in making some able-bodied people feel comfortable when talking to someone in a wheelchair. This often helps to set the stage for positive communication.

The following discussion will focus on three basic communication styles: assertion, aggression, and passivity. The general style will be described, followed by descriptions of specific behaviors that are typical of each style. Notice that these are behaviors, not words. It is how you say something (body language, tone of voice, etc.) that is important, not necessarily the words you use.

Assertion

Assertion involves standing up for your own personal rights. Express your ideas and feelings directly and honestly, but take into account other people's feelings, too. This involves respect—respect for you *and* respect for other people. To do this requires that you communicate clearly *and* that you ask what others might think and feel. In other words, cooperation and fair play are essential to being assertive.

In assertive behavior, your body actions are consistent with the verbal messages and add support, strength, and emphasis to what is being said verbally. The voice is appropriately loud to the situation; eye contact is firm, but not a stare-down; body gestures that denote strength are used; and the speech is fluent—without awkward pauses—expressive, clear, and with emphasis on key words.

Aggression

Aggression involves standing up for your personal rights, but in a way that ignores others' rights. This is not an honest way to communicate. It is almost always inappropriate and may create strong, negative feelings, such as anger or disgust.

The usual goal of aggression is domination and winning, forcing the other person to lose. Winning is insured by humiliating, degrading, belittling, or overpowering other people so that they become weaker and less able to express and defend their needs and rights. The basic message is: "This is what I think—you're wrong for believing differently. This is what I want—what you want isn't important. This is what I feel—your feelings don't count."

In aggressive behavior, the nonverbal behaviors are ones that dominate or demean the other person. These include eye contact that tries to stare down and dominate the other person, a forceful voice that does not fit the situation, sarcastic or condescending tone of voice, and parental body gestures such as excessive finger pointing.

Passivity

Passivity involves violating your own rights by failing to express honest feelings, thoughts, and beliefs. Expressing your thoughts and feelings in such an apologetic, self-defeating style may allow others to easily disregard you. The total message communicated is: "I don't count—you can take advantage of me. My feelings don't matter—only yours do. My thoughts aren't important—yours are the only ones worth listening to. I'm nothing—you are superior."

Passivity is nonassertion and shows a lack of respect for your own needs. It also shows a subtle lack of respect for another person's ability to take disappointments or to shoulder some responsibility. The goal of nonassertion is to appease others and to avoid conflict at any cost.

In nonassertive behavior, the nonverbal behaviors include avoiding eye contact, hand wringing, clutching the other person, stepping back from the other person as an assertive remark is made, hunching the shoulders, covering the mouth with a hand, nervous gestures that distract the listener from what the speaker is saying, and wooden body posture. The voice tone may be singsong or overly soft. The speech pattern is hesitant and filled with pauses, and the throat may be cleared frequently. Facial gestures may include raising of the eyebrows, laughs, and winks when expressing anger.

In general, the nonassertive gestures are ones that convey weakness, anxiety, pleading, or a self put-down. They reduce the impact of what is being said verbally, which is precisely why people who are scared of acting assertively use them. Their goal is to soften what they're saying so that the other person will not be offended.

RELAXING IN THIS STRESSFUL WORLD

Frequently, it seems there are too many things going on around you and no way to deal with all the daily hassles. Although no one can eliminate stress from your life, there are some ways of reducing the impact stress can have on your health. A great many health problems are directly linked to the strains of muscle tension, increased blood pressure, and increased heart rate that usually come along with stressful activities. Many people with spinal cord injuries say they find that the initial demands of rehabilitation are stressful. But even most able-bodied people you talk to will say that their days are often busy and stressful. This section offers two specific methods of dealing with stress: relaxation techniques and time management skills.

Progressive Relaxation

You cannot have the feeling of warm well-being in your body and at the same time experience psychological stress. Progressive relaxation of your muscles reduces pulse rate and blood pressure as well as decreasing perspiration and breathing rates. Deep muscle relaxation, when successfully mastered, can be used as an "anti-anxiety" pill.

Most people do not realize which of their muscles are chronically tense. Progressive relaxation provides a way of identifying particular muscles and muscle groups and learning the difference between tension and relaxation.

The following is a procedure for achieving deep muscle relaxation quickly. Whole muscle groups are simultaneously tensed and then relaxed. You may not be able to complete all the muscle movements, but do what you can. Repeat each procedure at least once, tensing each muscle group from 5 to 7 seconds and then relaxing from 20 to 30 seconds.

Remember to notice the contrast between the sensations of tension and relaxation. Try these exercises in a comfortable position (such as in a sitting position with your head supported), and practice at least twice a day until you have mastered these exercises.

1. Curl both fists, tightening biceps and forearms, pulling your fist toward your shoulder. Relax. Allow your arms to rest at your side.

2. Wrinkle up your forehead. At the same time, press your head as far back as possible, roll it clockwise in a complete circle, then reverse. Now wrinkle up the muscles of your face like a walnut: frowning, eyes squinted, lips pursed, tongue pressing the roof of the mouth, and shoulders hunched. Relax.

3. Straighten your back as you take a deep breath into the chest. Hold. Relax. Take a deep breath, pressing out the stomach. Hold. Relax.

Since some of the actions require neck and back movement, you need to get clearance from your doctor.

You may want to make a cassette tape of the basic procedure to improve your relaxation program. Remember to space each procedure so that time is allowed to experience the tension and relaxation before going on to the next muscle or muscle group.

Most people have somewhat limited success when they begin deep muscle relaxation, but it is only a matter of practice. Although 20 minutes of work might initially bring only partial relaxation, it will eventually be possible to relax your whole body in a few moments.

In the beginning, it may seem to you as though relaxation is complete. But although the muscle or muscle group may well be partially relaxed, a certain number of muscle fibers will still be contracted. Relaxing these additional fibers will bring about the emotional effects you want. It is helpful to say to yourself during the relaxation phase, "Let go more and more." Also, focus on deep breathing when you relax.

Time Management

This is another important way to deal with stress. When you leave the hospital after a recent injury, you will no longer have a staff member to help schedule your activities. For those of you working or returning to work for the first time after your injury, it is essential to develop skills in planning your daily routine. Parts of the following discussion were taken from *The Relaxation & Stress Reduction Workbook*, by Martha Davis, Elizabeth Eshelman, and Mathew McKay.

Time can be thought of as an endless series of decisions, small and large, that gradually changes the shape of your life. Inappropriate decisions produce frustration, lowered self-esteem, and stress. They result in the six symptoms of poor time management:

1. Rushing.

2. Always being caught in the middle of unpleasant alternatives.

3. Fatigue or listlessness with many slack hours of nonproductive activity.

4. Constantly missed deadlines.

5. Insufficient time for rest or personal relationships.

6. The sense of being overwhelmed by demands and detail and having to do what you do not want to do most of the time.

Time management techniques for relieving these symptoms have been developed by management consultants and efficiency experts who teach busy people to streamline their lives. Alan Lakein, who wrote *How to Get Control of Your Time and Your Life*, sees himself as a "time planning and life goals consultant." Many therapists, such as Harold Greenwald (author of *Direct Decision Therapy*), have also contributed to time management theory by developing techniques for facing and clarifying decision-making.

All methods of time management can be reduced to three steps:

1. You can establish priorities that highlight your most important goals and that allow you to base your decisions on what is important and what is not.

2. You can create time by realistic scheduling and the elimination of low-priority tasks.

3. You can learn to make basic decisions.

Before examining the three steps to effective time management, it will be useful to explore how you really spend your time. An easy way to do this is to divide up your day into three segments:

1. From waking through lunch

2. From the end of lunch through dinner

3. From the end of dinner until going to sleep

Carry a small notebook with you, and at the end of each segment (after lunch, after dinner, in bed just before sleep), write down every activity you engaged in and those that require assistance. Note the amount of time each one took. The total amount of time for all activities should be fairly close to the total number of hours you were awake.

Unless you are particularly interested in improving time utilization at work, simply describe work activity as socializing, routine tasks, low-priority work, productive work, meetings, and telephone calls.

Keep this time inventory for three days. At the end of three days, note the total amount of time spent in each of the categories. If you wish, you can divide by three to get the average daily time for each activity. You can also order the categories from the most to the least time-consuming to get a rough picture of your current obligations.

You should modify or add categories to suit yourself. You might wish to distinguish between conversation at home with intimates and talk at social gatherings or between shopping for pleasure and shopping for necessities. You may want to have specific categories for your daily self-care activities or just a general hygiene category. You might want to break down household chores into several categories. The important thing is to separate and examine categories of time use, and then determine if you want to spend more or less time engaged in each of these activities.

Setting Priorities

Having made your own time inventory, you can begin to compare your current use of time to important goals.

What did you want to accomplish in your life, what are you most proud of, and what might you most regret? Limber up your imagination and put anything down that comes to mind. Don't think about it or analyze it—if something occurs to you, write it down. Distill what you have written into your long-range goals.

Second, make a list of your one-year goals that stand a reasonable chance of being accomplished. Finally, put down all your goals for the coming month, including work priorities, improvement schemes, recreational activities, etc.

You have created three lists of goals: long-, medium-, and short-range. Deciding which are the top-, middle-, and bottom-drawer items can prioritize each list.

1. *Top drawer:* those items ranked most essential, most desired.
2. *Middle drawer:* those items that could be put off for a while but that are still important.
3. *Bottom drawer:* those items that could easily be put off indefinitely with no harm done.

Breaking Priorities Down into Manageable Steps

Now it is time to break down the top-drawer items into manageable steps that can be easily accomplished.

You have goals to work on. They are your top priorities. Give them a month. Next month you will make a new list. Some goals will remain top drawer, others will drop off. The goals will always be accompanied by a list of specific steps. Set aside a certain time period each day to work on your top-drawer goals. Emphasize result rather than activity. Try to accomplish one step toward your goal each day, no matter how small that step may be.

If you are a very busy person or one who finds it hard to keep focused on top-drawer items, you will need a daily "to-do" list. The to-do list includes everything you would like to accomplish that day. Each item is rated top, middle, or bottom. If you find yourself doing a bottom-drawer item when some of the tops are not yet finished, you can be almost certain that you are wasting your time. Work your way down. When the top items are completed, get to the middle-drawer tasks. Only when everything else is done should you permit your time to go to the bottom drawer.

You will find that it is often possible to just ignore the bottom items. They may never be missed. In making and following your to-do list, it is useful to be aware of the 80-20 rule: 80 percent of the value will come from only 20 percent of the items.

It is easy sometimes to let top-drawer goals slip to the back of your mind and say, "Not today. I'll get to it after I get the house cleaned up." One solution to this tendency is to make signs describing your current top-drawer goals and post them conspicuously around the house or office. Every time you look at them you'll be reminded of your priorities.

Making Time

There are four "must" rules and nine optional rules for making time. The four must rules are as follows:

1. Learn to say "no." Unless it's your boss who asks, keep away from commitments that force you to spend time on bottom-drawer items. Be prepared to say, "I don't have the time." If you have trouble saying no, see the section in this chapter on assertiveness training.

2. Banish bottom-drawer items unless you have completed all higher priority items for the day. Bottom-drawer items can wait.

3. Build time into your schedule for interruptions, unforeseen problems, unscheduled events, etc. You can avoid rushing by making reasonable time estimates for activities and then adding on a little extra time for the inevitable problems.

4. Set aside several periods each day for quiet time. Arrange it so that you will only be interrupted in an emergency. Focus on deep relaxation, using the techniques presented in this chapter.

Listed below are the nine optional rules for making time. Check three of them that would be most helpful to you. Begin the habit of following the rules you have marked right now.

1. Keep a list of short five-minute tasks that you can do any time you are waiting or are between things.

2. Learn to do two things at once. Organize an important letter in your mind while driving to work, plan dinner while vacuuming.

3. Delegate bottom-drawer tasks. Give them to your children, your secretary, your housecleaner, and your mother-in-law.

4. Get up a half hour or an hour earlier.

5. Watch less television.

6. When you have a top-drawer item to do, block off your escape routes:
   - Schedule daydreaming for a later time.
   - Stop socializing.
   - Put away the books.
   - Put away tiny, unimportant tasks.
   - Don't run out for ice cream or other sudden indulgences.
   - Forget the errands you could probably do more efficiently later.

7. Cut off nonproductive activities as soon as possible (e.g., socializing on the phone when top-drawer items are begging to be done).

8. Throw away all the mail you possibly can. Scan it once and toss it.

9. Stop perfectionism. Just get it done. Everyone makes mistakes.

INDEPENDENT LIVING

Is there life beyond the hospital walls?

Yes, there is a life beyond the hospital walls, and independent living is a way to approach your day-to-day life in society. Independent living means being in charge of your life and taking responsibility for your actions. Independent living is *how* you live your life, not *where* you live. For example, some people think that being alone in an apartment is independent living. It is independent living only if the person freely chooses that lifestyle based on his or her individual physical, social, and financial needs and on the available resources. For other people, independent living means choosing to reside in a nursing home. In the following paragraph, July Gulliom explains her choice to live in a nursing home.

A lot of people seem to feel that if they end up in a nursing home, that's the end of life and they will never see daylight or any of their friends again. One of the facts about a nursing home is that it's one of the most efficient mechanisms for getting an unwieldy body attended to....I have a full-time job and heavy volunteer activities. If I had to devote a lot of time to administering a mini-institution on my own behalf, I wouldn't be able to do what I want to do. I don't choose to spend my time that way....

The nursing home has a lot of space and a lot of staff, and the economies of scale make a lot of difference when they mean that you're able to come and go as you please. If I arrive at two o'clock in the morning, there are people waiting to put me to bed. I really

could not afford to hire someone to sit in my own house and do that for me.

How you make decisions about your equipment needs is another good example of independent living. Some people prefer to use equipment for assistance with tasks ("high-gadget tolerance"). Other people like the physical and mental challenge of doing difficult tasks, or they may prefer to limit their equipment ("low-gadget tolerance") and use "people power" when they need some help.

REMEMBER: Free choice means making a decision based upon:

- Your needs
- What you would like to happen
- The resources available to you

SOCIAL SURVIVAL TACTICS

A person with a spinal cord injury needs social survival tactics because:

- You are a member of a minority group in our society.
- You will run into negative stereotypes that people have about wheelchair or crutch users.
- The general public will notice you.
- You will be dealing with agencies and bureaucracies more than the average American will!

Social survival tactics are the tools you use to get the services, emotional support, and physical help you need. Some tools, such as the social skills of time management and assertiveness, have already been discussed. Other tools for survival and independent living include how you think through the social decisions that you face most frequently. This section will present some ways to solve basic social questions.

Social Decisions

Social decisions are crucial to your physical future. There are no right answers to these questions. It all depends on personal goals, and these goals can change throughout your life. Remember that these decisions are the foundation for your social and emotional survival. Listed below are two important questions.

- Where will I live?

- Will I live alone or with someone?

You will need new or different social skills to get what you want and need. Meeting new people after your spinal cord injury is really no different from before your injury. Be yourself, make eye contact, and talk sports, weather, or whatever you used to talk about.

Once you become aware of the particular social challenges that your disability may create, you will learn how to handle them. There are two major approaches to meeting these challenges. First, decide if you have the necessary basic social and communication skills that everyone needs. Second, decide if you need some special skills for dealing with common reactions to your disability.

These approaches help you think about yourself as a person first and then as a person who happens to have a disability. Many social challenges, such as finding a sexual partner, meeting new people, and wanting to be more assertive, are common to all people. Some challenges, such as having a waitress ask your companion, "What does he want to eat?", are directly related to having a disability. More often than not, the challenges you encounter

can be resolved by learning general social skills (assertiveness, how to handle anger). The special skills related to your disability can include how to deal with the nondisabled population.

Be an Effective Communicator

People with disabilities need to understand the thinking and actions of nondisabled people. At times their actions and reactions are frustrating and difficult to understand. All communication involves two parties, and miscommunication involves two parties. When an interaction or communication is not working, you need to ask two important questions:

1. Am I using my best and most effective communication skills?

2. Are the other people miscommunicating out of a lack of information or a lack of effective communication skills?

If you are using your best skills, go to question two. If the answer to question two is that the others lack information, then you need to educate them. If they are poor communicators, then it is their problem. People with disabilities often think the actions and words of nondisabled people are cruel and intended to be degrading when, in fact, the nondisabled people may just be ignorant, not cruel. They mean well but need suggestions for more helpful ways to interact with people who happen to have disabilities.

When you are doing your best and things are still not going well, the situation may call for special skills and understanding that relate directly to your disability. For example, you must judge when and how to discuss your disability with new friends and potential employers. These skills are learned by experiencing the situations first hand, consulting other people with disabilities, and by learning (reading) about the stereotypes of the nondisabled population to find effective, useful, and productive ways of overcoming those stereotypes.

It is not always an easy task, but being a member of a social minority group often requires that you become a teacher of the general population. You didn't ask for that role, but it does come with your wheelchair, crutches, and other paraphernalia. Learning these skills can result in increased self-determination and self-pride!

YOU CAN WORK IF YOU WANT TO WORK

Work is a significant part of our lives. It affects us so profoundly, both socially and psychologically, that many people identify who they are by their job titles The other aspects of their self-description (a father, a husband, an organizer) are often secondary. A job can affect how we perceive our status in society. "Oh, I'm just a _____." It influences the kinds of people with whom we associate. For many of us, our work is our life. The degree of satisfaction you get from your work directly affects the quality of the rest of your life.

Having had a spinal cord injury, you may be asking, "Can I work? What kind of job could I do?" The answer is: *YOU CAN WORK IF YOU WANT TO WORK*. W. Mitchell (who became paraplegic in 1975) says, "The way I look at it, before I was paralyzed, there were ten thousand things I could do; ten thousand things I was capable of doing. Now, there are nine thousand. I can dwell on the one thousand, or concentrate on the nine thousand I have left. And, of course, the joke is that none of us in our lifetime is going to do more than two or three thousand of these things in any event."

If job exploration and continuing your education interest you, you should meet with a vocational rehabilitation specialist.

FAMILY AND FRIENDS

When an acute spinal cord injury occurs, those people close to you are most likely to be as emotionally shaken up by your injury as you are. They may feel shock (numbness), disbelief, sadness, and anger as they see you move from surviving your injury through your rehabilitation process.

Their reactions may be quite familiar to you, or they may be very unexpected. You may or may not be able to understand the hows and whys of their reactions and actions. In any case, try to remember that this sudden change for you was just as unexpected and unwanted for them. Give yourself and them some time to adjust and think about all of these changes. Some tips on how to help both you and your family and friends during this time of transition follow:

- Try and talk about how all of you feel. By bringing it out into the open, no one has to guess how everyone else is taking it, especially YOU! They love you, and you love them, and that's not a bad place to start.

- Since your close friends and family may be afraid to bring up the subject for fear of causing you or them more pain, you may have to start the ball rolling. It will be hard, but it may be best in the long run. Timing is very important, however. Adjustment is a healing process, so trust your gut instinct in dealing with certain issues. If either you or your close ones aren't ready to discuss something, let it go for a little while. There will come a time in the natural course of adjustment when you will both feel right about it.

- Try not to hide all of your feelings. You don't have to be strong for your family and friends. This only makes it harder for them to talk with you.

- Also, remember that your family and friends are part of society and may have the same misconceptions and attitudes about people with disabilities. When you're able to, try to talk to them about this. You need to teach them the truth. Soon enough, you'll find them educating their friends and families too!

- If your family lives close to an SCI center, they may want to attend a family support group. Check the bulletin board for day and time.

- Sometimes, family and friends go overboard trying to do just about everything for you. For some people with disabilities, this becomes a smothering experience. For others, this is merely what they always expect from their close ones. This type of behavior may be O.K., or it may get tiring for both you and your family and friends.

- Figure out how and with what you'd like to have help. If your family and friends are doing too much, talk to them about it. Let them know how it makes you feel and why you'd prefer that they not do so much for you.

After you live with spinal cord injury for a period of time, the feelings you now have about your injury may be very different from those you experienced when you were first injured. You may be more comfortable with this change in your body and what you need to do to keep it healthy.

As you became more experienced in getting around town (either by car, van, public transportation, or wheelchair), you may have gained a new sense of freedom as well. These challenges have helped you learn and adapt to this new way of life.

Adapting to life with a spinal cord injury is a unique experience. Each individual does it in his or her own way. Whatever way you have chosen is O.K., as long as it keeps you healthy, both in mind and body.

Your family and friends have also adapted to your spinal cord injury. Many have come to realize that you are still the same person they've always loved except for some physical changes. Unfortunately, a few may not have been able to adjust to the new physical you, no matter how much they love you. Some people just can't. Relationships change in everybody's life, no matter if you're disabled or not. Being a spinal cord injured person is a challenging experience that offers a potential for growth.

BEING A PARENT

You can be a parent if you decide you can or want to be a parent. Many feelings and a great amount of thinking will contribute to that decision. Common feelings may be uncertainty about your ability to provide the physical care and financial support. Fear may arise about how a child will respond to you now that you are in a wheelchair. You may experience feelings of depression or discouragement that cause you to wonder about caring for another person. Or you may experience great joy and satisfaction as you realize your children need and respond to your caring and attention. You may be surprised how accepting and adaptable children are.

As you review your feelings and thinking, it is good to remember that bringing up children is a tough job and that every parent can feel uncertain at one time or another. Although your injury may change how you physically care for a child, it does not create insurmountable barriers. There are many adaptive tools, techniques, and even books that you can explore. Consult your rehabilitation team members for ideas.

When you are making changes because of a spinal cord injury, your child should be included in the process. If you are absent from the home due to a hospital stay, your children, of whatever age, need to have the absence explained at their level of understanding. You and your children need to know that a physical limitation need not change your relationship. Research has shown no difference in emotional and social development between children whose parents have a spinal cord injury and those who don't.

It is also important to remember that your rights as a parent don't change after a spinal cord injury. Custody of your children or your right to seek adoption cannot be denied solely on the basis of your disability.

Specific Thoughts to Keep in Mind

- Include your children in your rehabilitation program. Find out about visiting hours and passes out of the hospital with your family.

- Introduce your children and spouse to other parents with SCI. Have your children talk with their children.

- Include your children in family meetings in and out of the hospital.

- Continue the discussions with your children about your injury or related feelings after you leave the hospital. Seek out community counseling services that are recommended by your SCI social worker or psychologist.

- You can also work closely with your rehab team members about parenting concerns.

Deciding to Become a Parent

As a first step, you may wish to explore your physical capability to have children. Check with your SCI urologist and doctors. You may wish to consult with your social worker or psychologist if you are thinking about becoming a parent. If you discover you are physically unable to have children, consider adoption or artificial insemination. Take a look at the chapter on "Sexuality." It may also provide some helpful information about your options.

SOCIAL AND LEGAL RIGHTS

Exercising Your Legal Rights and Responsibilities

People with SCI are entitled to the same constitutional rights as all other U.S. citizens. In addition, many federal laws support the legal rights of citizens with disabilities in the areas of vocational rehabilitation, education, transportation, accessibility, social and medical services, tax exemptions, and Social Security benefits. Each individual state has various legal rights that are guaranteed. This section identifies some of the major federal laws and shows how you, the voter and the consumer with disabilities, can exercise your rights in a knowledgeable and responsible way. We will start with some general guidelines on how you can assert your rights and get the best results.

Be an Assertive Citizen

1. Know your basic rights!
2. Vote.

3. Keep a record of your transactions with agencies and programs. A file folder for each agency or program is a good idea. Include the following information:

   • Date.

   • Who you talked to.

   • Copies of letters, applications, and other paperwork.

4. If you think your rights have been violated, ask to talk with a supervisor, the administrator, or the person at that agency in charge of grievances relating to civil rights.

5. Learn the appropriate channels for complaints within the particular agency, local and state government, etc.

6. It is your responsibility to:

   • Be assertive, not aggressive.

   • Learn the established steps for civil rights complaints.

   • Listen.

Major Laws and How They Relate to You

There are a number of laws that exist and work for you. (*See table 13.A.*)

The Rules of Laws

Federal and state legislatures are elected and then pass laws that affect the lives of citizens.

After a bill is passed and becomes a law, regulations are written. These regulations state how agencies, businesses, and citizens will carry out the laws.

Regulations are the rules of our governmental system and directly affect our daily lives. For example, the regulations issued for the Americans with Disabilities Act (ADA) are detailed requirements that greatly affect both the public and the private sector. Hardly a person in America is unaffected by the need to comply with this federal statute.

When regulations are not properly followed or you think the regulations do not ensure the rights that you are guaranteed by law, then you can resort to legal action. The court system is set up to uphold laws and prevent unconstitutional regulations.

Americans with Disabilities Act (ADA)

In 1990, the Americans with Disabilities Act was passed, the most significant piece of civil rights legislation since the mid-60s. The ADA is a comprehensive ban on both public and private discrimination against people with disabilities. The five titles of the ADA cover employment, state and local governments, public accommodations, telecommunications, and miscellaneous provisions.

The law itself and regulations issued by five federal agencies are very specific as to certain requirements. The Department of Justice, the Department of Transportation, the Equal Employment Opportunity Commission, the Federal Communications Commission, and the Architectural and Transportation Barriers Compliance Board have all published regulations to implement the ADA and provide technical assistance to help people apply the law. The Internal Revenue Service provides two special tax incentives for businesses, one a tax deduction for any business to remove barriers, the other a tax credit for small businesses to comply with the ADA.

The following are the activities affected by the titles of the ADA.

Title I (EMPLOYMENT). No employer with more than 15 employees can discriminate against a qualified person with a disability in

TABLE 13A. Laws that Affect People with Disabilities

YEAR	PUBLIC LAW #	TITLE OF LAW	KEY PROVISIONS
1968	90–480	Architectural Barriers Act	Requires that buildings built with federal funds or leased by the federal government be made accessible.
1970	91–453	Urban Mass Transportation Act	Requires eligible local jurisdictions to plan and design accessible mass transportation facilities and services.
1973	93–87	Federal and Highway Act	Requires that transportation facilities receiving federal assistance under the act be made accessible; allows highway funds to be used to make pedestrian crosswalks accessible.
1973	93-112	Rehabilitation Act	Prohibits discrimination against qualified handicapped people in programs, services, and benefits that are federally funded; creates Architectural and Transportation Barriers Compliance Board.
1975	94–173	National Housing Act Amendments	Provides for the removal of barriers in federally supported housing; establishes Office of Independent Living in U.S. Department of Housing and Urban Development to serve disabled people.
1978	95–602	Rehabilitation Comprehensive Services and Developmental Disability Amendments	Establishes independent living as a priority for state vocational rehabilitation programs; provides federal funding for independent living centers.
1980	96–265	Social Security Disability Amendments	Removes certain disincentives to work by allowing disabled people to deduct independent living expenses in computing income benefits.
1984	98–435	Voting Accessibility for Elderly and Handicapped Act	Provides for access to polling places and ballots and all activities related to voting.
1986	99–435	Air Carrier Access Act	Prohibits discrimination on the basis of disability in the provision of air transportation.
1988	100–430	Fair Housing Amendments Act	Prohibits policies that discriminate on the basis of disability in housing; requires newly constructed multifamily housing to provide accessible units.
1990	101–336	Americans with Disabilities Act	Extends to people with disabilities civil rights similar to those available through the Civil Rights Act of 1964.
1999	106-170	Ticket to Work and Work Incentives Improvement Act	Provides vocational, employment, and health-care supports to people on SSDI and SSI who want to work.

any area of employment. This includes hiring, promotion, fringe benefits, sick leave, etc. An employer must make reasonable accommodations to enable an individual with disabilities to perform the essential functions of a job, unless the accommodation causes an undue hardship.

Title II (STATE AND LOCAL GOVERN-MENTS). State and local governments and all departments, agencies, and instrumentalities must ensure that their programs are accessible. These requirements apply to all parts of all state and local governments, regardless of whether they receive federal funds. The most important implication of this section is the creation of ADA coordinators for most governmental agencies. When consumers encounter disability barriers, they can now obtain information and advice from an individual who is required to be knowledgeable about disability issues.

Buses used in public transportation must be equipped with lifts; paratransit must be provided to individuals with disabilities that are unable to use the established fixed-route system.

Title III (PUBLIC ACCOMMODATIONS). The coverage in Title III affects almost all private businesses, services, and agencies. A place of public accommodation is a facility operated by a private entity that falls within one of the following categories:

- Place of lodging, such as a hotel
- Establishment serving food or drink
- Place of exhibition or entertainment, such as a theater or stadium
- Place of public gathering, such as a convention center or auditorium
- Sales or rental establishment

- Service establishment, such as a bank, dry-cleaner, offices of lawyers, doctors, or accountants
- Station used for transportation
- Place of public display or collection, such as a museum or library
- Place of recreation, such as a park or zoo
- Place of education, such as private schools
- Social service establishment, such as a senior center, day care center, or homeless shelter
- Place of exercise or recreation, such as a gym or golf course

Places of public accommodation must remove architectural and communications barriers where it is readily achievable to do so. All new construction is to be accessible.

Private entities that provide transportation services must, depending on the circumstances, acquire accessible vehicles or provide equivalent service to individuals with disabilities. This means that if it is relatively easy and inexpensive to take out a barrier, it must be done. Barriers include steps, narrow spaces, lack of TDD phone service, or a policy prohibiting a waiter from reading a menu to a visually impaired person. If barrier removal is an undue hardship, each entity has an identified ADA appeal process.

Title IV (Telecommunications). This title of the ADA reformed the national telephone system to include people with hearing and speech impairments. Providers of telephone service must provide "relay" service. Relay operators are middlemen in conversations between individuals using TDDs (telephone device for the deaf) and people using regular phones.

Title V (Miscellaneous). Title V provides that the Architectural and Transportation Barriers Compliance Board (the Access Board) will issue guidelines to ensure that facilities and vehicles are accessible to individuals with disabilities.

Section 504 of Rehabilitation Act

Section 504 and its regulations prohibit discrimination against any qualified person on the basis of his or her disability by an entity that receives federal funding. The regulations apply to every program of the federal government. Three very important areas covered by Section 504 are education, employment, and community services.

Ticket to Work and Work Incentives Improvement Act of 1999

The Ticket to Work program is a new approach to providing vocational services with an emphasis on customer choice of providers. It is designed to increase flexibility and will begin in some states starting in 2001, with full implementation set for 2004.

The Work Incentives Improvement Act extends Medicare Part A (Hospitalization) benefits, without any premium payments, from the current 3 years to 7.5 years. The law gives state Medicaid programs the option to provide coverage for people with disabilities who are working. Both of these programs are scheduled to take effect October 1, 2000.

Expedited reinstatement of Social Security benefits after leaving work status and a new policy of not allowing medical review of cases when a person using the Ticket to Work program returns to work are two new features of this Act. These changes are scheduled to take effect January 1, 2001.

There are some other grants and demonstration projects included under this Act. The purpose is to have more services for working people with disabilities and encourage federal agencies to grant tax credits and other employment incentives so more persons with disabilities will enter the workforce.

Getting an Education

Post high-school educational programs and institutions must provide reasonable access to admission exams, classrooms, testing, student housing, and support services. In some instances on-site assistive devices may be provided by the educational institution.

OPTIONS FOR HEALTH CARE AND FINANCIAL PLANNING

Advance Care Directives

Advance care directives, directives to physician, and living will are all terms used to describe the same basic document. The formats for these documents may be different from state to state or hospital to hospital. They are all for the purpose of helping you take control of the scope and type of health care you want in life-threatening situations if you can't communicate your desires to your doctor. Hospitals and other care facilities are required to inform you about the option of establishing advance care directives. Do not resuscitate orders and durable power of attorney for health care are two other ways to communicate your health-care wishes. The following is an explanation of each.

A Do Not Resuscitate Order takes effect after you have talked with your doctor and your doctor has written the order. It is an order written by your doctor while you are in a hospital or nursing home that directs the staff NOT TO DO cardiopulmonary resuscitation. When there is no doctor's order, then full resuscitation will occur. Some states, such as Washington, allow you to prepare a directive of Do Not Resuscitate that can be used by emergency personnel in the community. Ask your health-care provider if this option is available in your state.

An Advance Care Directive takes effect when you are unable to communicate. It is a document drafted by an attorney and signed by you that lets you specify your particular desires about health-care procedures you may and may not want done if you are not able to communicate.

A Durable Power of Attorney for Health Care takes effect if you can't communicate. It is a document drafted by an attorney and signed by you that identifies a person who will make decisions on your behalf about health care procedures and treatment plans. You need to show this person your advance care directives and discuss your health-care wishes.

OPTIONS FOR ANOTHER PERSON TO HANDLE YOUR MONEY

There may come a time when you need for another person to help you manage your money. Often the terms used to describe this process are confusing and unfamiliar. Some states may have variations in the names of these procedures, but they are generally the same things. Remember, always consult an attorney if you feel you need legal help.

Power of Attorney

This is the paperwork signed in the state where you reside giving someone else the authority to manage your money. It can include giving the power to sell property. This type of paperwork means you and the other person can both do your business. You are sharing this power, not giving it away.

Veterans Administration Fiduciary

This is an internal VA process whereby a professional documents that you can't handle your money. VA appoints an official to handle your VA money and, possibly, your other income from government sources. The fiduciary has the control of your money.

Court Appointed Guardian of Estate (Money)

This is a court procedure where a professional signs papers saying you are unable to handle your money. The court then appoints someone to handle your money; you don't control your money.

Court Appointed Guardian of Person (Social and Health Decisions)

This is a court procedure where a professional signs papers saying you are unable to make decisions about your medical care or social well-being (that you are "a danger to yourself or others"). The court appoints someone to make decisions for you. This has nothing to do with your money.

GETTING COMMUNITY RESOURCES

The most effective methods for getting the community resources you need are the following:

• Be assertive

• Consult your peers

• Remember patience and a smile are highly effective when dealing with stressed-out bureaucrats

• Know your legal rights

To find local resources, contact information and referral agencies, vocational rehabilitation agencies, or your state's liaison to the President's Committee on Employment of Persons with Disabilities.

RESOURCES

Publications

Depression: What You Should Know: A Guide for People with Spinal Cord Injury
Purchase:
PVA Distribution Center
P.O. Box 753
Waldorf, MD 20604-0753
(888) 860-7244
www. pva.org.

The Americans with Disabilities Act: Your Personal Guide to the Law
Purchase:
PVA Distribution Center
P.O. Box 753
Waldorf, MD 20604-0753
(888) 860-7244
www. pva.org.

Anatomy of an Illness as Perceived by the Patient. N. Cousins. Bantam Doubleday Dell Publishers, 1991.

The Relaxation & Stress Reduction Workbook. M. Davis, E. Eshelman, and M. McCay. New Harbinger Publications, 1998.

Social Relationship and Interpersonal Skills: A Guide for People With Sensory and Physical Limitations. M. Dunn. Institute for Information Studies, Fairfax, VA, 1981.

A New Guide to Rational Living. A. Ellis and R. Harper. Wilshire Book Co., 1997.

Don't Say Yes When You Want To Say No. H. Fensterheim and J. Gaer. Dell, 1975.

Direct Decision Therapy. H. Greenwald. EDITS, 1973.

When Bad Things Happen to Good People. H. Kushner. Avon Books, 1994.

How To Get Control of Your Time and Your Life. A. Lakein. Signet, 1973.

When I Say No I Feel Guilty. J. Smith. Bantam, 1985.

Contact: The First Four Minutes. L. Zunin and N. Zunin. Balantine, 1975.

Web Sites

www.usdoj.gov/crt/ada/adahom1.htm
The Americans with Disabilities Act home page within the Department of Justice's web site, this site links to ADA technical assistance materials, DOJ's information line, status reports, enforcement information, and more.

eeoc.gov
The site of the Equal Employment Opportunity Commission provides information on laws, regulations, and policy guidance regarding employment.

www.dol.gov/odep
The Office of Disability Employment Policy offers information, training and technical assistance on employment issues as well as links to the Job Accommodation Network (JAN), providing information about job accommodations for people with disabilities.

Chapter 14

Sexuality is much more than what happens between two people in bed. When we talk of sexuality, we are not just talking about gender (male or female). People's sexuality is shown in many ways such as the way they present themselves in interactions with others, clothing, their body image, hobbies and interests, and in their grooming habits. Sex, on the other hand, is the physical interaction of two people. It may or may not be a very intimate experience. It may or may not be with someone of the opposite sex. It does, however, express sexuality.

For many spinal cord injured people, male or female, the change in or loss of genital sensation is one of the biggest impacts on sexuality. Many spinal cord injured people say that sex is much more intimate and spiritual than it was prior to their injury (instead of orgasms being just physical and focused on the genitals, they can be more a state of mind). These people have found much pleasure in discovering their own and their partners' bodies in new ways. They do so from touching, caressing, and exploring each other. This intimacy and pleasure requires open and willing communication. This means talking about what feels good, how and where to touch, or things like bladder and bowel function. Having ongoing discussions related to sexual functioning helps both the person with SCI and the partner to know what to expect.

In the past, the assumption was made that people with SCI were no longer capable or interested in sex. Today, we know this is not true. It is now recognized and increasingly accepted that sex, marriage, and being a parent can be a part of anyone's life (this means with or without a disability). A physical disability does not eliminate sexual feelings. Individuals with SCI experience the same sexual feelings as do individuals without SCI.

You can lead a sexually active life, and you can maintain intimate relationships if you choose to do so. This chapter will provide information to help you accomplish these goals. The topics to be covered include myths and misconceptions about sexuality and disability, anatomy of sexual functioning, changes in sexual functioning after SCI, and effects of SCI on fertility and pregnancy (both male and female).

MYTHS AND MISCONCEPTIONS ABOUT SEXUALITY AND DISABILITY

Myth: It is not appropriate for health-care providers to discuss sex with patients.

FACT: Sex is a natural part of life. It deserves attention in your rehabilitation program. Sex and sexuality are health issues and should be discussed between you and your health-care providers.

Myth: People with disabilities are no longer sexual beings.

FACT: We are all sexual beings. This does not change after spinal cord injury.

After you are discharged from the hospital, you may find that people on the outside don't react to you in the same way they did before you were injured. You may also find that new people you meet may seem a little uncomfortable or anxious around you. They may not know what to say or how to relate to you. You may not be seen as a sexual person or a potential sex partner. For a time just after your injury, you may react to yourself in the same way. This is because many people simply do not see that people with disabilities are still sexual beings.

If you already have a sex partner, you may notice that he or she does not approach you sexually in the same way as before. Likewise, you may be somewhat timid about initiating sex with your partner. If you are, it may come from fear and anxiety about being able to perform sexually with a "new" body. You may not know how to begin or what to expect. That can be very frightening. Spinal cord injury sex education is one way to start working out those fears. This, along with good social and communication skills, can help fix this situation.

The onset of paralysis will likely affect your genital function. This does not erase your ability and desire to sexually please and be pleased. Through education, exploration, and experimentation, mutual satisfaction is again possible. You will get to know your body much better than you did before you were injured. You will also likely learn how to do some sexual acts in new ways. This is discussed in more detail in the next section.

Myth: Marriage and parenting are no longer options for people with SCI.

FACT: People with spinal cord injuries do fall in love. Marriage often follows. Men and women who are spinal cord injured do have success in bearing children and keeping happy households.

In the long run, the effect of spinal cord injury on your sexuality has a lot to do with how you feel about yourself (self-esteem). Your skill and confidence in close relationships make up part of your ability to function sexually. You must accept yourself as a sexual being and use your learned skills. You need to explore your body for sensation, movement, and reaction. To successfully guide your partner, you need to know the territory. In doing so, you can obtain sexual satisfaction for yourself and your partner. Keep in mind that:

- The presence of spinal cord injury does not mean the absence of desire or romance.

- Inability to move does not mean inability to please or be pleased.

- Absence of sensation does not mean absence of emotions.

- Loss of genital function and/or sensation does not mean loss of sexuality.

ANATOMY OF SEXUAL FUNCTIONING

This section will identify and describe areas of the body involved in sexual functioning.

The Male Sex Organs
(See figure 14.1.)

- *Scrotum (SCRO-tum):* A sack of thin muscle and skin that houses and protects the testes.

- *Testes (TESS-teez):* Egg-shaped organs that produce and secrete the male sex hormone testosterone (tess-TOSS-ter-own) and produce sperm.

- *Epididymis (epp-i-DID-i-miss):* A storage place for sperm.

- *Vas Deferens (VASS deaf-air-ENNS):* One of the narrow tubes through which sperm travels to exit the body.

- *Seminal Vesicles (SEM-i-null VESS-ick-ulls):* Two small glands that add fluid to the sperm.

- *Prostate Gland (PROSS-tate gland):* A small gland shaped like a walnut that adds fluid to the sperm to make semen. This gland is found just below the bladder. The urethra passes through it.

- *Ejaculatory Duct (ee-JACK-you-lah-tor-ee duckt):* A small passageway in the urethra through which semen (SEA-men) (both the fluid and the sperm) moves close to the time of ejaculation.

- *Cowper's Gland (COW-purrs gland):* Two pea-sized glands that secrete a small drop of fluid after a man becomes sexually excited to lubricate the urethra.

- *Urethra (your-EETH-rah):* A tube that is a passageway for the sperm to exit the body during ejaculation. It also carries urine out of the body.

- *Penis (PEA-nis):* The organ that contains the urethra through which sperm and urine pass. It becomes erect during sexual stimulation and, when hard, penetrates the vagina during sexual intercourse.

The Female Sex Organs

(See figure 14.2.)

- *Labia Majora (LAY-bee-ah mah-JORR-ah) ("Large lips"):* The larger of the skin folds that surround and protect the vaginal area.

- *Labia Minora (LAY-bee-ah min-ORR-ah) ("Small lips");* The smaller skin folds found inside of the larger ones. These lie directly beside the vaginal opening.

- *Clitoris (CLITT-or-iss):* The organ located just above the urinary opening and just below where the tops of the labia minora meet. It is made of the same type of tissues as the penis. Unlike the penis, the only purpose of this organ is for sexual excitement.

- *Vagina (vah-JINE-ah):* A tube leading from the labia to the uterus. The penis is inserted into the vagina during sexual inter-

FIGURE 14.1. The Male Sex Organs

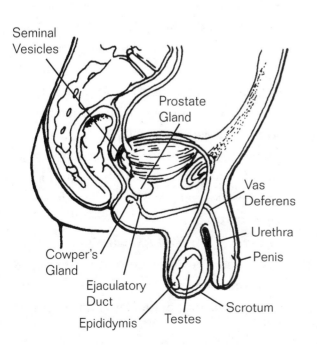

FIGURE 14.2. The Female Sex Organs

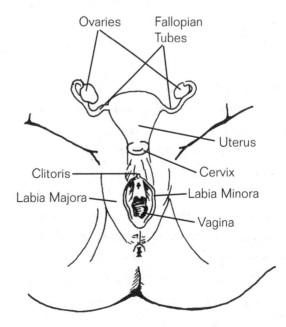

course. During childbirth, a baby passes through the vagina from the uterus.

- *Cervix (SURR-vix):* The opening into the uterus from the vagina. Through it, sperm enters to fertilize an egg and a baby exits to be born.

- *Uterus (YOU-turr-uss):* A thick hollow muscle located in the lower abdomen. Its purpose is to carry and nurture a child.

- *Ovary (OH-va-ree):* Two small organs that take turns every month to produce eggs. They also produce the female sex hormones, estrogen *(ESS-tro-jin)* and progesterone *(pro-JESS-turr-own)*.

- *Fallopian Tubes (fall-OPE-ee-an toobs):* Two tubes that are attached to the top of the uterus. On the outer ends of the tubes are finger-like pieces of tissue that catch the eggs from the ovaries and pass them down the tube to the uterus. For the most part, it is within these tubes that eggs are fertilized by sperm.

SEXUAL FUNCTIONING AFTER SCI

If you have some or no feeling below the level of your injury, you may wonder what sex will be like now. It's true that genital sensation is ONE (but only ONE) part of the sexual experience, but you still can feel full sexual sensations above the level of your injury. This includes your ears, neck, face, and mouth.

Areas that are particularly sensitive and produce sexual arousal are called erogenous zones. Many people with SCI discover that areas other than the genital areas and nipples are sexually exciting when touched. Use them and also your other senses to heighten these feelings with the help of the largest sex organ of all—your brain. Sexual function requires a fine-tuned coordination of different parts of the nervous system. Think about people working together as a team on some goal. When some team members don't do what they are supposed to do, the result may be that the goal is only partially achieved or not achieved at all. The same thing happens in spinal cord injury: some nerves cannot do what they used to do.

In males, the changes after SCI are typically in erection, ejaculation, and orgasm or climax. The lack of, or decrease in, feeling and movement may also change the sexual experience. In women, changes in sexual function include decreased ability to lubricate and orgasm.

Male Sexual Function

Erections

There are two types of erections: psychogenic and reflexogenic. Each involves different parts of the spinal cord. The degree to which each one is affected depends upon where and how complete or incomplete your injury is.

- *Psychogenic (SIGH-ko-JENN-ick) Erections.* These erections occur from sexually related thoughts (fantasy), seeing a good looking person, looking at erotic pictures, reading sexually exciting material, or hearing sounds that are sexually stimulating. If your SCI is in the lower lumbar or sacral area and is incomplete, you may be able to have a psychogenic erection. If you have an incomplete injury above the T12 level, psychogenic erections may still sometimes occur.

- *Reflexogenic (re-FLEX-o-JENN-ick) Erections.* These erections occur through a reflex mechanism in the sacral part of your spinal cord. Your brain plays no part in getting this type of erection. All you need is an intact functioning reflex system at S2, S3, or S4 segments of the spinal cord. This is present in cervical, thoracic, and lumbar (upper motor neuron) spinal cord injuries. Any type of stimulation to the scrotum, penis, or anus may cause this type of an erection. Perhaps you've noticed this when you wash or apply your condom catheter.

If you have a reflexogenic erection, it is important to remove the sexual stimulation after you and your partner are finished. If not, the penis can remain erect for a long time, which can cause some medical problems.

If having a partial or full erection is not easy and you feel it is a major part of your sexual activity, you do have some options. See the section on "Adaptive Equipment and Medications to Enhance Male Sexual Functioning" for a discussion of options. Feel free to discuss these options with your physician or other rehabilitation team members.

Ejaculation

Ejaculation is the mechanism that allows semen to be discharged. In normal ejaculation, muscle contractions cause spurts of semen to be forced outward from the penis. Part of the process that allows normal ejaculation is closure of the *bladder neck* so that semen can flow past the bladder and out of the urethra. In many spinal cord injured men, *retrograde ejaculation* occurs. This happens when the bladder neck stays open and semen travels the easy, shorter pathway into the bladder rather than the long distance out of the urethra. *(See figure 14.3.)*

If you have an incomplete injury, you're more likely to ejaculate than those men with complete injuries. But, some complete spinal cord injured men can ejaculate a good deal of the time. The best way to check out your ejac-

FIGURE 14.3. Ejaculation

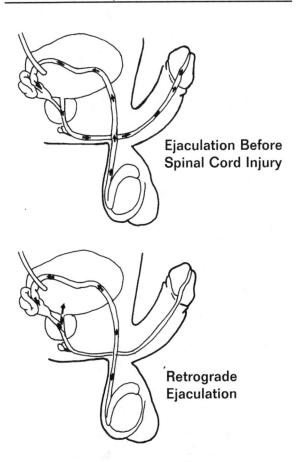

Ejaculation Before Spinal Cord Injury

Retrograde Ejaculation

ulatory status is to try it out. Be patient: give yourself a few chances to see if this system still works.

Orgasm

Orgasm is the pleasurable sensation generally associated with rhythmic contractions of the perineal muscles and the base of the penis. It may also be a psychological means of achieving pleasure, as in the absence of tactile sensations or loss of ejaculation.

Female Sexual Function

Lubrication and Arousal

In women, lubrication of the vagina works the same way as erections do in men. An injury to the sacral part of the spinal cord may result in lack of lubrication. An injury above this level may leave reflex lubrication intact. With an upper motor neuron (UMN) injury, stimulation to the genitals and vagina will most likely cause this reflex. You may also have psychogenic lubrication if you were injured around or below the T12 level of your spinal cord. For women who are not able to lubricate, you may wish to use a water-soluble jelly to enhance lubrication. It is not advisable to use vaseline or any oil-based product or any perfume-based material because these do not dissolve in water and can become a source of infection.

Orgasm

Orgasm is the culmination of sexual excitement. There is little information regarding orgasm in women with SCI. This is an area of continued interest and investigation.

ADAPTIVE EQUIPMENT AND MEDICATIONS TO ENHANCE SEXUAL FUNCTIONING

Male

Vacuum Pump

Vacuum erection/constriction devices are the least invasive and least expensive of current treatment options. The devices produce an erection by creating a vacuum around the penis, which triggers blood flow into the corpora cavernosa. The erection is maintained by using a tension band or ring placed around the base of the penis. Although this method seems fairly simple, it is very important to receive "hands on" instruction with your practitioner. Preparation requires viewing a video and reviewing written information.

Penile Injections

This choice involves giving a shot into the penis about 20 minutes before sexual activity. Alprostadil is the FDA approved drug used in injection therapy. The dose of Alprostadil is individualized and therefore testing and training are necessary. It is very important for the man or his partner to feel comfortable about his receiving a shot into the penis (corpora).

Transurethral Therapy (MUSE)

This is a urethral suppository (Alprostadil). There are very specific instructions needed to use this form of therapy. It is important for you to receive training for this form of therapy.

Viagra (Silendafil Citrate)

Viagra is the first FDA approved oral agent for erectile dysfunction. Viagra helps restore penile blood flow and erection in response to sexual stimulation. Once again, it is important that you receive instructions about this medication. Viagra is ABSOLUTELY contraindicated in patients using medications that contain nitrates in any form.

Penile Prosthesis

These are silicone rod devices implanted in the penis that have fluid chambers to simulate a true erection. An important consideration for patients and partners is that this is an invasive procedure (surgery) and is considered irreversible. All other feasible options should be investigated prior to discussion of penile implant surgery.

Final Note

In order for any treatment to be successful, it is advisable to include your partner in information and learning sessions.

Female

The overall quality and quantity of information concerning sexual functioning for women with SCI are poor. Most discussions are centered on bowel and bladder management, with some emphasis on return of "normal menstruation" and the need for protection if sexually active.

Women are interested in learning how to achieve sexual satisfaction when sensation is lessened or gone. Self stimulation or the use of vibrators can enhance sexual discovery or rediscovery. Questions often asked are related to "how can I have a satisfactory and fulfilling sexual experience?" Answers and solutions often come about through personal exploration or work with a partner. There are currently many research projects underway that are studying sexual functioning of women in general. One study is currently investigating the use of Viagra in enhancing sexual arousal.

The area of sexual functioning with women who have a SCI is open for much discussion as well as further research investigation. Communication with your provider will keep you up-to-date on improvements and new findings.

SCI AND INTIMACY

Compared to before your SCI, sexual activity now requires some planning, and the idea of spontaneous sex may change as well. Many people like spontaneity and the freedom to explore themselves and their partner. This can happen if the time is taken to explore your new self, both in body and mind. Your healthcare provider may have suggestions as well as more reading material.

Things to Think About Before Sexual Activity

Preparation will enhance and not destroy the moment.

Autonomic dysreflexia (AD). In some individuals, sexual activity can cause episodes of AD. You need to be able to recognize AD, know how to treat it, and be prepared. See the chapter on "Autonomic Dysreflexia."

Bladder Management. If bladder control is a problem or concern and you have planned in advance a certain time for sex, decrease your fluid intake three to four hours before sex. Emptying your bladder just before sex is the best insurance against incontinence. Catheters and other urinary equipment may be removed prior to sex. It is your choice. If you do not wish to remove them, listed below are some things to consider.

- You can use longer connective tubing with a larger volume "night" bag. This will allow for a bigger area of movement. Check once in a while to make sure the tubing is not pinched or kinked.

- Men can bend a foley catheter against the shaft of the penis and place a condom over it. If this is done, extra lubrication may be needed around the tubing coming into contact with the penis. This will prevent chafing of the skin.

- If you wear an external (condom) collecting device, you may wish to remove it. However, some people prefer to remove their catheters before sex and replace them after sex. You, your partner, or attendant will need to be taught catheter change. Have the supplies ready to replace the catheter following sexual activity.

- Women not wishing to remove their foley catheter will often tape the tubing to their stomachs or upper thigh area.

- If you have an ostomy, extra tape may be needed to help prevent the chance of leakage. Avoid direct pressure against the ostomy bag, if you can. This also helps prevent leakage.

- If you have a suprapubic catheter, tape the tubing out of the way. Be sure to use a tape that will not pull on your skin.

Leakage and accidents are not the end of the world. They can happen even with all proper preparation and planning. People without spinal cord injuries sometimes have problems with incontinence too. You may want to place a waterproof pad over your mattress. It may also be helpful to keep towels around the bedside in case of accidents.

Bowel Management. To avoid accidents with your bowels, plan ahead for your bowel care. You may want to do it in the morning or just before intercourse so that it will not be a problem.

Preparation as Foreplay. Making a bath or shower part of foreplay can certainly be fun. It can help take care of unpleasant body odors as well.

If you require assistance to transfer, position, undress, or handle hygiene, you may need to include your attendant, caregiver, or partner to prepare for sexual activity. These activities can always be made a part of foreplay. Positioning yourself for sex will be your choice. It will also vary with the type of sexual activity in which you wish to engage. Check with your practitioner, physical therapist, or occupational therapist for any possible limitations in positioning.

Surroundings. Sexual activity is always better in a setting that is comfortable for both of you. Think about your surroundings. Where are you most comfortable having sexual activity (e.g., your wheelchair, a bed, couch, hotel)?

Environmental barriers may limit accessibility for sexual activity. For example, a person with SCI may have an accessible residence but a partner's residence may not be accessible.

Spasticity. Some people use spasticity to help heighten sexual pleasure. In some cases, spasticity can be used to obtain an erection. Leg extension or spasticity may increase the sexual experience.

Spasticity can also be a hassle during sex. Spasticity can prevent certain sexual positions. Your best bet is to maintain your range of motion as outlined by your therapist. During your therapy process, you may also learn to position and move your body in ways that will minimize your spasticity.

Diseases. Sexually transmitted diseases (STDs) can affect sexually active individuals with SCI as easily as anyone else. Always practice safe sex. In particular, any activities that involve the exchange of blood or semen may place you at risk of contracting the AIDS virus. Use of a condom will decrease the risk. You can contact your health-care provider, the local AIDS hotline, or Department of Health for more information. If you notice any abnormal discharge or any abnormalities of the skin on your genitalia, consult your health-care provider for an examination.

FERTILITY AND REPRODUCTION

Pregnancy—The Male Perspective

If you can ejaculate or have any mucus-like fluid from your penis during sexual activity, you will need to use birth control if you do not want your partner to get pregnant. Any fluid from the penis could contain sperm. The ability to impregnate a woman varies with each man. However, two problems are common in males with SCI: inability to ejaculate and poor semen quality. Semen samples can be obtained and analyzed at many major medical centers. It doesn't matter if you can ejaculate or not as techniques exist to assist ejaculation. If you cannot ejaculate or can but have not been successful in getting your partner pregnant, referral to a specialized urology clinic for further evaluation is possible. These clinics can conduct an analysis of your fertility (the ability to father children). Specialized procedures can be used to retrieve sperm that can then be inseminated into a partner. Many issues regarding fertility and reproduction are handled by these specialty clinics.

Vibratory stimulation to produce semen is accomplished with specially designed vibrators that have adjustable frequency and amplitude. Education on the procedure is done in the clinic, as well as the first trial. This provides semen for analysis. Thereafter, people with SCI at T7 or below can carry out the procedure at home to get semen for insemination. Training includes recognition of ovulation in the partner to make conception more likely.

Electroejaculation. Electroejaculation involves using a rectal probe to apply electrical stimulation that causes ejaculation to occur. These techniques can be used to obtain samples to be tested for fertility or used for artificial insemination. Sometimes several samples are combined to increase the quality of the sperm so that there is a greater chance of success of insemination procedures. If you are interested in more specific information, talk to your practitioner and a referral will be made if appropriate.

Artificial Insemination. Artificial insemination is the introduction of sperm into the vagina or cervix by artificial means. Sperm that was collected by vibratory stimulation or electroejaculation can be used in this proce-

dure to increase the likelihood of fertilization. Prior to artificial insemination, both male and female fertility may be tested. If a couple desires children but the sperm of a male is of poor quality and cannot be used, another option is artificial insemination with the sperm of a donor. This will require a referral to a specialty center.

Adoption. Adoption is another alternative for anyone who desires to have and raise children. Adoption agencies and programs can help you decide if it is the right choice for you. These programs can also inform you about legal procedures. Both married and single people can apply for adoption. You cannot be discriminated against because you are a person with a disability. If you feel you have been denied these services because of your disability, treat this situation the same as any other case of discrimination. See the chapters on "Community Resources" and "Psychosocial Adjustment" for more information.

Pregnancy—The Female Perspective

It may take spinal cord injured women up to a few months following injury to have a period (menstruate) again. Once menstruation returns, pregnancy can occur. If you don't want to get pregnant, you'll need to practice birth control. You should discuss all birth control options with your practitioner.

Artificial insemination and adoption are also options for women with spinal cord injuries who desire to raise children. See the discussions above in "Pregnancy —The Male Perspective."

When you are pregnant or considering becoming pregnant, talk with your gynecologist about special medical considerations related to your spinal cord injury.

SEXUAL COUNSELING

These services are a response to the growing number of people, disabled or not, who want to know more about their sexuality. Sexual counseling is now available for individuals or partners. Seeking professional advice or counseling is not always easy to do but you should focus your attention on obtaining as much information as you feel you need. There are different kinds of counseling for different problems.

Most major medical centers have these services available. Various SCI organizations as well as the internet may be able to help you identify services in your local area. The guidance below will make it easier for you to find the help you need.

Getting Started

On the whole, the most difficult part of the process is bringing up the subject and saying what the problem is. Don't get discouraged!

Is the problem related to genital function? This includes changes in your ability to have or keep an erection or in vaginal lubrication. If so, consult your urologist.

Is the concern more related to a sexual relationship, lack of one, or a desire to feel better about your sexuality? Your practitioner or local mental health center will be able to counsel you or refer you to a counselor in your community.

If you are concerned about your ability to become a biological parent, you will need to speak to a fertility specialist.

Finding a Good Counselor

While you were in an SCI unit, you could get counseling on most sexual issues from the SCI team. Counseling is also there for you through the SCI outpatient clinic, specialty clinics within the hospital, or another agency in your community. You may be purchasing their services. A smart consumer needs to know what he or she is buying. Here are a few good questions to ask the counselor. Remember, the type of individual(s) you need to see, such as a therapist, urologist, fertility counselor, will depend upon the issues or concerns you are seeking assistance for.

- How much experience do you have in sexual counseling?
- What type of training or professional degree have you received?
- Have you worked much with clients who have disabilities?
- How long will I need to see you and how much will it cost?

If the counselor has little experience, ask:

- Do you have an interest in working with clients who have disabilities?
- Would you be willing to consult the SCI service for more information about spinal cord injuries?

Some sexual counselors may not have experience with clients who have disabilities. This doesn't mean that they are not good at what they do. More to the point is their willingness to uncover facts about spinal cord injuries when they are needed.

Not all sexual concerns are due to your disability. Sexual and relationship problems can occur in anyone's life!

One way to get practical information about the issues discussed in this section is to talk with other people with disabilities. Some communities provide peer support groups or independent living centers. These can help you find a peer who has found a way of sexually adapting to a disability. Your SCI team may also be a source of information about resources in your community.

Books, magazines, pamphlets, and web sites are also ways to obtain information. Examples of sources are listed below but this list is by no means comprehensive. Web sites may also contain references as well as links to other web sites.

RESOURCES

Publications

Sexuality After Spinal Cord Injury: Answers to Your Questions. S. Ducharme and K. Gill. Brookes Publishing Co., Baltimore, MD, 1996.

Reproductive Issues for Persons with Physical Disabilities. S. Haseltine, S. Cole and D. Gray. Brookes Publishing Co., Baltimore, MD, 1997.

Women with Physical Disabilities: Achieving and Maintaining Health and Well-Being. D. Krotoski, M. Nosek and M. Turk. Brookes Publishing Co., Baltimore, MD, 1996.

Web Sites

www.sexualhealth.com
Dedicated to providing access to sexuality information, education, counseling, therapy, medical attention and other resources for individuals with disabilities.

Every community has a number of services and programs available to help you and your family. That's what is meant by the term "community resources." Depending upon where you live, these services may be provided by the state, county, or community. Your social worker may be able to guide you if you need assistance.

Due to the number of community resources available, it is helpful to think about a specific resource under a general area, for example, housing, financial programs, or transportation. Community resources in a number of these general areas will be discussed below. Under each area, a brief explanation will be provided, with general contact information.

Here are some tips for calling a community resource:

• Call at the beginning of the workday.

• Always write down the name, title, and phone number of the person who gives you information, as well as the content of your conversation and the date. If you still have questions, call the agency again to verify the information you have.

• Make up a note card of all your personal information, e.g., Social Security number, VA benefits, hospitalization dates, doctors' names, and family contact names and numbers. It's nice to have it organized, because you are going to have to report this information many times.

• *Be persistent.* If the line is busy, call again. If the person is out, leave a message. Keep calling until you get the information you need. Don't give up!

• Visiting the agency may get you the information you need more quickly. If you are unable to do this yourself, appoint a spokesperson or advocate to act on your behalf. You may even want to visit the agency with your spokesperson.

INFORMATION AND REFERRAL SERVICES

An information and referral service provides general information over the telephone free of charge. This is done confidentially, so you can ask whatever you'd like without having to identify yourself.

This type of service offers information about all the programs in general that are available in your area. Ask if the program in which you are interested includes disabled individuals. Let them know what your disability is when you discuss your specific need. This will really make clear *exactly* how they can accommodate you.

HOUSING

Accessible housing is of primary importance for individuals with physical disabilities. Such housing may need to include negotiable ramps, doorways, bathrooms, and, when possible, modified kitchen areas. In selecting a living arrangement, it is best to look for specific features to accommodate your wheelchair. See the chapter on "Home Modifications."

Housing Authorities

Housing authorities for low-income families, low-income elderly, or low-income physically disabled people exist in many counties and towns. The waiting lists for low-cost accessible housing may be very long (months to a year). Call your county or city housing authority to obtain an application and to be put on the waiting list as soon as possible. When your name reaches the top of the waiting list, you can always say you don't need it, if that is the case. Financial eligibility is based on a national formula. Many low-paid working people qualify. If you qualify, the basic payment formula is approximately one-third (1/3) of your income.

Section Eight (8)

Rental Assistance Program funds are available to aid eligible individuals and families in lowering their monthly rental cost by paying a portion of it. Eligibility is based on gross annual income. The program utilizes existing housing and, for the most part, the applicant must find the housing and negotiate with the landlord.

Housing Assistance Organizations

Programs are available in certain areas to help individuals locate housing. Be sure to call an information and referral agency about accessible housing.

VA Specially Adapted Housing for Veterans

This is a program designed to pay some of the costs in purchasing a house. Eligible veterans with a service-connected disability who meet other requirements may receive a VA housing grant. The grant can only be used once. Contact your local VA regional office to apply.

VA Home Improvement or Structural Alterations

This program is designed to pay for some of the cost of remodeling your own house or a rental. Any eligible veteran may receive funds for major structural alterations and home improvements that comply with specific guidelines. Contact your local VA regional office or medical center.

Independent Living Programs

Some independent living programs provide transitional housing as well as peer counseling, advocacy, transportation, recreational activities, and more. Check with your social worker or the website resources at the end of this chapter about the independent living programs in your area.

VOCATIONAL SERVICES

Vocational rehabilitation services are available through federal and state government programs if you are eligible. Vocational rehabilitation services have different names throughout the United States, such as the Department or Division of Vocational Rehabilitation (DVR), rehabilitation services, or vocational rehabilitation. Your vocational rehabilitation counselor can best explain the many services that the DVR can provide. Some of the services may include:

- Medical, psychological, and/or vocational evaluations to help with job planning. Appropriate treatment can be authorized as well as equipment to aid in DVR programs.

- Counseling and guidance to achieve your rehabilitation plan and employment goal.

- Vocational education in college, trade school, or commercial school, and on-the-job training.

- Maintenance and transportation funds while you are pursuing vocational goals.

- Job placement assistance and follow-up to determine that the job is suited to your highest capabilities.

VA Vocational Program

VA administers programs for education and training for eligible veterans. Seek out the vocational counselor at the nearest VA spinal cord injury center to determine your eligibility for VA vocational rehabilitation programs and general education or training.

HOME HEALTH NURSING SERVICES

Maintaining your health is up to you. However, help may be available through the county or city public health department, the Department of Veterans Affairs, and nonprofit nursing services (for example, Visiting Nurse Services). These agencies have health professionals who may come into your home and help you with care needs on a limited basis, if you meet age and income restrictions.

Many hospitals have hospital-based home care or SCI home care programs that can send staff into homes depending upon geographical location and insurance coverage. The cost of the service and who pays for it are different for each agency. In addition, physician's orders are usually needed to obtain services. Consult with your social worker or your local public health department for names of agencies.

FINANCIAL ASSISTANCE

The loss of income after a crisis like a spinal cord injury can be a major worry. Specific programs are available for individuals with a financial need and a medical disability. A general outline of the federal and state programs follows.

Federal Financial Programs

Social Security Administration (SSA)

The SSA operates the program of Social Security Disability Insurance (SSDI), Supplemental Security Income (SSI), Medicare, and Retirement and Survivors Benefits. Call the national toll free number at (800) 772-1213. It may take several months to get your first check.

In applying for SSDI, SSI, Medicare, or Retirement and Survivors Benefits, keep in mind that *referrals and applications can be taken over the telephone.* You do not need to apply in person, and a family member or representative can apply for you.

- *Social Security Disability Insurance* may provide a partial income for individuals who have been employed and are now disabled. There is up to a seven-month waiting period before benefits begin.

- *Medicare,* a federal government health insurance program, is available to recipients of SSDI after two years of receiving benefits.

- *Supplemental Security Income* provides some income to people in financial need without regard to past work experience. Eligibility is determined on the basis of income, age (over 65), resources, and your disability. If you receive SSI, you will also be eligible for Medicaid Health Insurance through the state.

Know the Social Security rules and guidelines and keep up to date! Call the toll free number, check your annual Social Security statement, and visit the Social Security web site.

State Assistance Programs

State assistance programs are run through offices known as the departments of social services, health and social services, welfare, or human services, to name a few. The financial criteria for income and Medicaid benefits can vary from state to state.

Many programs may be available to you or your family. Call your County Department of Social Services if you need help with the following services.

Medicaid

Medicaid is a state-operated program for low-income people. It provides medical coverage for hospitalization and treatment; homemaker, home health aide, and visiting nurse services; transportation related to medical needs; and equipment. The services vary from state to state.

Food Stamps

Food stamps allow people with low incomes to buy more and better food. If you are eligible to participate, you pay a certain amount of money each month, and receive food stamps of a higher value. That gives you a bonus each month to spend at grocery stores for food and staples.

Aid to Families with Dependent Children

This program is designed to provide financial assistance and benefits to families with dependent children who are in need. Financial assistance provides money to help with purchasing of food, fuel, clothing, utilities, personal needs, and shelter.

Chore Services/Attendant Care

This program helps individuals living in their own homes by providing essential housekeeping or personal care. This monthly cash grant could be paid to you as an employer of an attendant or chore-worker, or it can be paid to an agency under contract to provide services to you. Some states have different administrative structures for housekeeping (chore services) versus personal care (attendant care services). Contact your local, county, or city department of social services. Each state has its own eligibility requirements, some of which are very restrictive.

Workers' Compensation

This state-regulated program provides employees injured on the job with health care, weekly income payments, and rehabilitation services.

Financial support and coverage by workers' compensation is in conjunction with insurance company support and coverage. It is ordinarily much more substantial than other state-supported financial programs.

To be eligible, an employee must incur a disability while working for an organization with worker's compensation coverage. Each company contracts with its own insurance company and, as a result, *individual benefits can vary.*

Further information may be obtained through your state department of labor and industries, workers' compensation, or industrial commission. The name of workers compensation agencies varies considerably, so contact your employer's human resources or personnel department.

Department of Veterans Affairs Assistance Programs

People with disabilities who are veterans may be eligible for benefits including hospitalization, medical treatment, educational programs, pensions, and other federal programs.

In addition, a state veterans service office may be available in your city or town (usually in the city hall). Under extreme circumstances, they can provide emergency financial assistance.

You can look in the phone book blue pages for the Department of Veterans Affairs offices nearest you.

A veterans benefits counselor will be available to speak with you while you are in a VA SCI center or as an outpatient of a VA SCI clinic.

EMPLOYMENT

For many people with SCI, employment is a significant part of their lives not only for financial freedom, but also for self-satisfaction. The ADA prohibits discrimination in employment on the basis of a person's disability.

Government agencies help promote equal hiring opportunities. The federal Office of Personnel Management conducts a rigorous action program to ensure hiring of people who have disabilities. Other sources of employment information and assistance are the state department of employment security, Federal Job Information Center, and VA vocational counselors. Seek our your vocational counselor for more specific information.

MENTAL HEALTH COUNSELING SERVICES AND CRISIS INTERVENTION

Community health centers, family service agencies, or centers for independent living can provide crisis intervention and counseling when difficulties arise. Consult with your social worker or psychologist or community

mental health center and keep in mind these general guidelines:

- Consider the experience and training of the individual providing counseling services. Pay special attention to their experience with people who have spinal cord injury or physical disabilities.
- Discuss your expectations for counseling sessions. This may include concerns to be discussed, number of sessions, and cost.
- Ask if the counselor is willing to consult with your doctors and others on your rehabilitation team.

ATTENDANT SERVICES

If you need an attendant to help with your personal care and household maintenance, programs are available to pay for these services. A variety of funding sources and methods of attendant management have been set up by different funding sources. National Medicaid policy has increased the options for state attendant care programs. Consult your local Medicaid agency. See the chapter on "Attendant Management" for more information.

LEGAL ASSISTANCE

Local Legal Aid Services

Most communities throughout the United States offer sliding-scale legal aid services. This means that the cost to you is determined by your ability to pay. If you are unable to locate the address of your community legal aid office, contact your state bar or law association, and they will refer you to the office nearest your home. Also, many law schools offer free or low-cost legal services.

Information and referral services can help you locate a lawyer.

Protection and Advocacy Systems

The federal government has mandated a system in each state and territory to provide protection of the rights of people with disabilities through legally based advocacy. These Protection and Advocacy Systems (P&As) were established to address public outcry in response to the abuse, neglect, and lack of programming in institutions for people with disabilities. Congress has created distinct statutory programs to address the needs of different populations of people with disabilities.

What Can You Do?

You can become more active in the disability movement to help people with disabilities by working together with other people with disabilities who share your views. Changing the system requires strength in numbers. Keep in touch with other consumer organizations around the country to learn what they are doing.

Federal programs and policies can influence many of the issues surrounding the disability community. Activists should bring these issues to the attention of nondisabled consumers and reform groups to add strength to their organization through the political and public media. *You can become knowledgeable, and you can get involved!*

TRANSPORTATION

Travel always requires planning—when you have a disability, it just takes more planning. Almost all modes of transportation are accessible to people who use wheelchairs, but it's worth double checking to avoid surprises.

When making your arrangements, be certain to ask the right questions. What services can you expect from transportation personnel? Is there a charge for a attendant/personal assistant? Do not assume that policies are consistent among transportation providers or that they will remain unchanged. Ask these questions each time you make a reservation.

Finally, the key to success in any traveling you do is good planning. Develop a travel plan that covers all aspects of your personal needs, e.g., comfortable clothing, time requirements, proper bowel and bladder scheduling, meals, transfer techniques and tools, who (such as airline or train personnel) might need information, and easy access to medication. Make your travel plan part of your trip and you will be happy you did.

Public Transportation

For getting around town, many public transit vehicles are now wheelchair accessible. Call your transit system to see if it is fully accessible; if not, they will accommodate you by putting an accessible vehicle on your route or by paratransit. If you are eligible for paratransit with your home transportation system, other cities must honor that eligibility while you visit—but be sure to notify them of dates of travel and check for any restrictions. Project ACTION keeps an updated website about accessible public transportation in many locations around the United States. Taxis are not required to be accessible under the ADA, but in many cities accessible cabs are available. Check the Project ACTION web site or your local chamber of commerce.

Air Travel

Under the Air Carrier Access Act, discrimination on the basis of disability is prohibited.

Carriers must have policies in place and training programs to ensure that airline personnel know what is required. For instance, passengers who have a foldable wheelchair and pre-board may stow their wheelchair in an onboard closet if it does not displace other passengers' luggage already in the closet. You may want to keep your wheelchair cushion with you. Using your cushion on the airplane seat may help to protect your skin during the flight. Be safe, do pressure releases.

Carriers are responsible for assistance in boarding and deboarding, in helping you make connecting flights, and returning your mobility equipment to you in the same condition that you released it to them. They will **not** help with personal care either at your seat or in the bathroom. You will almost certainly be boarded by a boarding chair, a narrow chair that carrier personnel can maneuver down an airplane aisle. Half of aisle seats on new planes must have movable armrests; in older planes, you may have to transfer over an armrest. Be very assertive in asking for assistance and telling carrier personnel the manner by which to assist you.

If you cannot assist in your own evacuation of the plane in case of emergency, you must bring (and pay for) your own assistant. If the airline determines that you require such assistance, and you disagree, the airline will provide passage for the assistant, but they may choose the assistant, perhaps an airline employee. That person is responsible for assisting only in the case of evacuation. If you do travel with an assistant, the airline must provide you with seats next to each other on the plane.

Be aware that airline personnel will not provide personal assistance on the plane. They will help in boarding, information, stow-ing luggage, and helping you get to and from the bathroom; they will not assist within the bathroom or with eating.

Amtrak

Amtrak has a special program that offers discounts for rail passengers with disabilities. Amtrak personnel will help with boarding, information, and at-seat services such as delivering meals, stowing luggage, and getting to and from the bathroom. They will not assist in eating, personal hygiene, or providing medical services en route. Amtrak's publication, *Access Amtrak*, will inform you of Amtrak services for travelers with disabilities.

Greyhound

Assistance is available from Greyhound to passengers with disabilities. At this point, very few Greyhound buses are wheelchair lift-equipped. You must call Greyhound ADA Assist Line at (800) 752-4841 at least 48 hours before your departure to arrange for a lift-equipped bus. You will be asked for information to help Greyhound personnel provide the assistance you need. If you cannot provide prior notification, Greyhound will make every reasonable effort to accommodate you without delaying bus departure schedules.

With some restrictions, personal care assistants may travel free on Greyhound. The ADA Personal Care Attendant ticket will be issued only to the personal care attendant, only at the time of travel, and only for one-way.

Tour Buses

While all tour-type bus services are covered by the ADA, they are allowed to phase in new lift-equipped vehicles. Therefore, you must call ahead of time to make arrangements, whether you are taking a tour or a regularly scheduled bus trip.

Rental Car Travel

All rental car companies must provide cars with hand controls. Contact the rental companies one week in advance.

Ship Travel

Even foreign-flagged ships operating in U.S. ports are covered by the Americans with Disabilities Act. However, standards for compliance have not yet been developed. Generally, the bigger a ship is, the better the chance of it being accessible. There are mixed reports on the crew's availability to help. Contact the shipping line for more information. Ask if they have an ADA coordinator (a person in charge of ensuring compliance with the Americans with Disabilities Act). See below under Hotels and Motels, for questions you may want to ask.

HOTELS AND MOTELS

Hotels and motels are covered by Title III of the ADA. While most hotels have accessible rooms, you still need to ask the right questions, e.g., how wide is the doorway to the bathroom, are there grab bars and a hand-held shower, are shower chairs with back rests available. Don't just take at face value the statement that the room is accessible—if it doesn't work for you, it isn't.

RESOURCES

Publications

New Horizons: Information for the Air Traveler with a Disability

Purchase:

Department of Transportation
Aviation Consumer Protection
Division, C-75
400 Seventh Street, SW, #4107
Washington, DC 20590

Download: http://airconsumer.ost.dot.gov/publications/horizons.htm

The ADA: Your Personal Guide to the Law

Purchase:

PVA Distribution Center
P.O. Box 753
Waldorf, MD 20604-0753
(888) 860-7244

www.pva.org

Web Sites

www.access-able.com
Access-Able Travel Source is dedicated to aiding travelers with disabilities and mature travelers with practical information needed to go across town or around the world.

www.amtrak.com/plan/accessibility.html
This site contains tips from Amtrak about accessibility services and tips on making your travel as barrier-free as possible. Also on the site is information on routes, schedules, meals, and accommodations.

www.ctaa.org
Community Transportation Association of America's members are rural, small urban, and community-based transportation providers. This site provides information on accessible transportation in these areas.

www.fhwa.dot.gov/
This site provides links to Department of Transportation ADA regulations and enforcement and features information on the Air Carrier Access Act.

www.fodors.com
Fodors Travel Services is known as the web site destination for any destination. Search and book airline tickets, hotels, cruises, and rental cars.

www.frommers.com
Budget Travel Online
Arthur Frommer's budget travel on-line offers airfares, hotels, cruises, special hot spots of the month, long with tips and resources for all travelers.

www.gsa.gov/frs/firsuse.htm
Provides information about using the Federal Information Relay Service, which acts as an intermediary between individuals who hear and speak and individuals who are deaf, hard of hearing, or have speech disabilities, for nation-wide communications with and within the federal government.

www.greyhound.com
Visit this site for trip planning information and to learn about Greyhound's services for travelers with disabilities. Or call their ADA Assist Line at (800) 752-4841.

www.hud.gov
The U.S. Department of Housing and Urban Development site offers information on home buying and renting, fair housing laws, and accessibility issues.

www.projectaction.org
Project ACTION Accessible Traveler's Database is a comprehensive database that offers a listing of accessible paratransit services in the United States, supplemented with information on accessible tours, airports, private shuttles, and taxi services.

www.napas.org
Protection and Advocacy Centers are part of a federally mandated system in each state and territory that provides protection of the rights of people with disabilities through legally based advocacy.

www.ssa.gov
The official web site of the Social Security Administration. It posts recent news releases from the administrator's office about changes in Social Security benefits. The site also provides access to Social Security forms, laws, and regulations.

www.travelintalk.net
Travelin' Talk is a global network of people with disabilities who share knowledge about their hometowns.

Organizations

National Council on Independent Living
1916 Wilson Boulevard, Suite 209
Arlington, VA 22201
(703) 525-3406
(703) 525-4153 TTY
www.ncil.org

Centers for independent living are organizations that provide four core services for people with disabilities: systems and individual advocacy, information and referral, peer support, and independent living skills training. The goal of these centers is to create opportunities for independence and to assist individuals with disabilities to achieve their maximum level of independent functioning within their families and communities. They work to ensure physical and programmatic access to housing, employment, transportation, recreational facilities, and health and social services.

There's a lot to be said for having a reason to get up in the morning. Your job is one of those reasons.

For many of us, our whole journey through education has been focused on one career goal. For others, that career choice is still a little blurry, but we get by. And we enjoy doing whatever we can. Heaven knows, you don't have to be a career hound to find a job that meets your personal and financial needs.

There are three vital parts to job hunting. One is to figure out what you like to do. Then you find out what you can do. Last but not least, you assess what is out there that you can tap into.

WHERE TO START

Since your spinal cord injury, you may have started looking at your working life in a way you have not done before. This would include taking a second look at your job skills, possible job changes, and your interests. How did you get into the work you were doing before your injury? Did you select it or did it just kind of happen?

You may feel that since you were injured you have "lost" what you thought were important job skills. At what level is your injury? Has it caused you to lose some of the physical abilities that you had before? Well, don't short-change yourself! You still have many job skills. You have just come to take most of them for granted. You can still communicate, persuade, teach, negotiate, direct, or listen. And how about personal traits you have developed over the years? Are you friendly, empathetic, curious, assertive, imaginative, or practical?

When you are up to it, you need to begin thinking about what job skills and personal traits you do have that you *enjoy using* and feel you *do well*. You might even want to try learning some new job skills. You can accept those skills you have and work at building them up. Only then can you begin to explore *where* and *how* they can be used in the job market. But rest assured that before you can sell yourself to an employer, you must know your product...YOU. You might want to look at the chapter on "Psychosocial Adjustment."

HOW TO GET A JOB

Did you know...?

- Jobs in general: Ninety percent of these are not listed in want ads or with employment agents.

- Blue collar and white collar jobs: Sixty-three percent of these jobs are obtained through *options pursued by the job* seeker. They include contacts through friends and relatives.

- Professional, technical, and managerial jobs: Seventy-five percent of these are obtained through *personal contacts*.

In looking at numbers like that, it becomes clear that you need to keep your eyes *and* ears open for possible job options. You might even drum up a few of them on your own! Put a bug in someone's ear. Lots of businesses give their staff bonuses for bringing new talent to them to fill open jobs. You'd be doing your friends a favor in asking them if they know of jobs where they work. If you get the job, they get the bonus!

Need Some Help?

You may be one of those lucky people who has always known what you wanted to do. A spinal cord injury hasn't changed that. You may also be the type who knows exactly how to get what you want, too. You are a rare breed. Most of us, however, spend a major part of our work lives searching for the "right" job. We change jobs often as we test our skills and interests in different workplaces. Each time you have to make a job change, though, it is a huge task that none of us relishes!

Motivation to get out there into the field is always hard. This can be worse if you aren't even sure where to start. Try this: Set up a plan of attack, take a deep breath, and *JUMP*!!

That's all well and good, you say, but that's also not very realistic. I still don't know where to start. Can you give me more to go on?

To begin with, if you do well with self-motivated projects, there are many books and computer internet sites that will be useful to you. They provide a step-by-step approach to matching your chosen skills with a suitable job. Your public library may have many helpful resources. One of the best-known is the *Occupational Outlook Handbook*, which is updated regularly by the US Department of Labor.

Some of us, though, do better in career planning if we get personal help. That is the time when you should call on your vocational rehabilitation counselor. Whether you just want to discuss some career concerns or you are ready to start some serious planning, this staff member is prepared to help you.

VOCATIONAL REHABILITATION

Vocational rehabilitation can be a really good resource. Specialists in this field can help you with career planning. Vocational rehabilitation counselors and occupational therapists work together with you. They will help you assess your job interests and skills, academic abilities, personal traits, and physical capabilities. They can help you set career goals and define ways for you to achieve those goals. If you are ready to go to work, they can help you plan your mode of attack on the job market.

Vocational Counseling and Testing

Vocational counseling and testing are provided to help you with the tasks listed below:

- Assess your skills and interests.
- Develop an appropriate plan for returning to work.
- Get retraining.
- Find meaningful unpaid activity.
- Improve your job finding skills.

This may include a referral to the state division of vocational rehabilitation. If you are a veteran and have a service-connected disability, you may be referred to chapter 31 of the VA Vocational Rehabilitation Program. These are programs for further planning and financial assistance with retraining. During the first stages of your rehabilitation program, you may be referred to Occupational Therapy (OT) for *pre-vocational testing*. This looks at your job skills through the use of simulated work samples. You may be given a *Physical Capacities Evaluation*. This can help assess your physical ability to perform varied types of work.

Your vocational rehabilitation may also include a *work hardening program (or a pre-vocational job station program*, as it is sometimes called). This is a chance for you to work at a variety of real jobs to help you assess your job interests, skills, physical endurance, and work habits. The program is structured so that you begin working (on an unpaid basis) a few hours per week, depending on your own vocational needs. These hours may increase gradually as your rehabilitation schedule and physical tolerance allow.

There are many different state and federally funded *on-the-job training (OJT)* programs. If you are a service-connected disabled veteran, you can apply for on-the-job-training through the VA vocational rehabilitation program. These OJT programs often pay a part of your salary for the first few weeks of your employment. This is a nice incentive for the employer to hire you and give you training on the job! OJT programs can be a good way for you to develop job skills and gain work experience.

The Americans with Disabilities Act (ADA) is a law that was established to protect you from discrimination in hiring. You need to know your rights under this law when you start your job search.

Job site modification and equipment modification are also there for you. These programs help you become employable in a certain kind of job. The purpose of all of this is very simple. It is for you to find a job that you are good at and that you like. The faith you have in yourself will grow as you learn more about what you like to do and what you can do. Then, when you do start looking for a job, you will be able to show your best effort. You will find that you are hired by people who feel you can be of great value to the company.

Web Sites

www.dol.gov/odep
The Office of Disability Employment Policy offers information, training and technical assistance on employment issues as well as links to the Job Accommodation Network (JAN), providing information about job accommodations for people with disabilities.

Recreation! What images or ideas come to mind when you hear that word? Water or snow skiing? Camping? Catching a movie with a friend? How about playing basketball, gardening, or just reading a book?

Look at your life and think about all the recreation-activities you have done. Some you have enjoyed and have made a part of your day-to-day life, like exercising, playing cribbage, playing a musical instrument, or sewing. Others activities may cause you to wait in anticipation until the season or opportunity is there, such as snow skiing, rock climbing, fishing, or traveling. Each of us has a unique set of recreation or leisure interests. Simply, the recreation activities you do *REFLECT WHO YOU ARE AND WHAT IS IMPORTANT TO YOU!*

Leisure activities have many meanings in our life. Our recreation allows us to express ourselves, release tension, master skills, meet people, and improve our health. Furthermore, we need these activities to experience risk and challenges, be exposed to new ideas, experience accomplishments, and build pride. Most importantly, through our leisure we are able to relax and have fun! Each of us discovers these benefits in the recreation we choose to do. These activities become a menu of options that become your leisure lifestyle.

Remember that your leisure is something you freely choose to do. There are days when you fill your free time with a great deal of action. Then there are other days when you simply feel like laying on the couch and watching TV. That is okay. The intent of this chapter is to motivate you to feel the freedom of expressing your leisure time as you choose.

This chapter will provide information, answer questions, and identify resources that will assist you towards that goal.

BEGINNINGS

While you are in the hospital, you will have the opportunity to explore how leisure fits into your life. Recreation or leisure might be the last things on your mind right now. However, relax. There will be plenty of time. As you progress in your rehabilitation, you may have opportunities to participate in recreation or *recreation therapy* programs within the hospital and out into the community. Give them a try.

Programs within the hospital will allow you to enjoy an activity that you have an interest in. These will also be programs that are designed to support the skills or strengths that you are focusing on in the other therapies. Playing a Monopoly™ game with other patients or family or developing a hobby such as building car models can provide necessary stress relief and add some fun during a very difficult time. But these activities also can help build hand function, endurance, and other benefits that support your recovery. Give these opportunities a chance; recreation can really help.

Community activities are essential to your rehabilitation. The thought of going out of the hospital may seem very scary at first. These feelings are very important, do not minimize them. However, do not let these feelings stop you. You may have the opportunity to go out to eat, to the movies, to a sporting event, or perhaps home. These outings will help you discover your strengths, learn about accessibility, develop wheelchair skills, and have fun. The first outings may be difficult, but they will get easier.

One final note before we move on. Remember that your recreational interests are a part of you. Try not to cross important interests off your list because you think you cannot do them anymore. Give yourself time to heal and to get stronger. You will soon discover that what you think may not be possible right now, actually is. Be patient with yourself and don't give up!

GETTING INVOLVED

Step one is to figure out what is important. As we have stated, look back at your life and make a list of all the activities you enjoy doing. Include on the list recreation activities that you have also dreamed of trying, like scuba diving or flying. Again, avoid making decisions now about what you think is not possible. These options will show you what is important for you to make a part of your life.

The second step is to look at your strengths and areas that you may need support. Has your injury affected your mobility, the way you get around? Are you using a wheelchair, or perhaps a walker, a cane, or nothing at all? How much strength and coordination do you have in your arms and hands? Has your vision or hearing been affected? Are people available to provide assistance if you need it to participate in the activity? How have your endurance and stamina been affected? Talk with your therapists and doctors and get a clear idea. It is important for you to understand the extent of the impact that your injury has had on you. This way you know what skills to rely on and the others that need to be developed or worked around. Remember, life is a journey. You will discover new capabili-

ties along the way that you did not think were possible.

The final step is to just do it! The remainder of the chapter will discuss accessible recreation and resources. However, an important consideration is that the first time you attempt anything is the hardest. Initial comments and feelings from others in your position are that, "I can't do this anymore because I have a spinal cord injury." Or "I have done enough, I don't need to do it anymore." Write these feelings down. The first time that you try an activity that you have done for years like going to the movies, shooting skeet, playing billiards, or even playing ball with a son or daughter may be challenging at first. But keep at it. In six months, you can look back and congratulate yourself on how far you have come.

ACCESSIBLE RECREATION

Accessible recreation has come about from people like you wanting to be active and break down the barriers. Accessible recreation is simply making a leisure activity possible. This is accomplished through adaptive equipment and sometimes finding a new way to approach the activity.

Adaptive equipment helps an individual overcome limitations, such as altered mobility or hand function. If you enjoy downhill skiing, there are skis known as mono-ski or bi-ski. Which one you use will depend on your level of sitting balance, strength, and skill. A mono-ski is simply a ski designed with a bucket type seat with shock absorbers and a strut attached to a single ski. A person uses ski poles or poles that are modified to add grip or support. You may start out with an instructor tethered to you and work up to using the ski independently on the steepest runs. A bi-ski is designed for a person with less sitting balance and strength. The seat is similar, yet another ski is added at the base for additional support and stability.

The British Columbia Disabled Sailing Association of Canada was started by a group of people who wanted to sail. They developed a sailboat that can be modified for anyone who has a desire to sail independently. They have even designed controls that are completely hands free using sip-and-puff technology that interfaces with an autohelm. The individual is able to use the rudder, sail controls, and even an emergency radio. Skin protection is accomplished through just turning the boat or tacking. Once the person learns to sail, the level of injury doesn't matter. Success is measured on how well the person reads the wind.

Adaptive equipment is not designed to make an activity easier; it is to allow you to get involved. For example, people with quadriplegia who have a loss of strength and coordination in their arms and hands still enjoy hunting using lighter rifles, shooting stands, and trigger extensions. If their mobility is affected, hunters use 4-wheel all-terrain vehicles or horses to get into the backcountry. They find a way.

There are many types of sports wheelchairs. Basketball, tennis, and quad rugby wheelchairs are designed very similar to day-to-day wheelchairs. However, the position you play will determine the type of design you use. If you want to move fast but be able to turn quickly with more stability, you may choose a wheelchair with greater camber or angle of the wheels. There are sports frames that are lighter but stronger, making it difficult for someone to block you. Sports wheelchairs are also designed to support an individual's seat-

ing, posture, and skin protection, as your day-to-day wheelchair does, while allowing you to be competitive in that sport.

Sports have also become more competitive and accessible through equipment development and subtle rule changes. Tennis allows a person in a wheelchair an extra bounce and use of the doubles lines. Basketball teams are made up of a variety of individuals with different strengths. Each player is evaluated and given a rating. A team can put on the court at any time only players whose ratings add up to a certain point value. In this way, the team must coordinate each other's strengths while supporting each other. This way the teams are equal. Track and field have developed lightweight racers and throwing stands. This equipment allows athletes to go faster and accomplish more.

Know the extent to which your spinal cord injury has affected you. Challenge yourself to do as much as you can. If you enjoy bowling, try a regular ball, then a handleball or push stick before using a bowling ramp. Try an activity without any adaptive equipment first. You may find that you have more strength than you give yourself credit for.

To enjoy recreational activities, you do not have to recreate the wheel. There are many resources out there to provide information, equipment, and opportunities to help get you involved. How do you find this help? First, start a resource file of information that you discover. Write the information and contact numbers in an address book, develop a card file, or computer program. Keep track and update the information. Include information that you might not use until later or that may be helpful to someone else.

Where to look? You may be surprised to find out that resources may be just around the corner. Look in the Yellow Pages under Recreation. Contact your local YMCA or YWCA, community centers, parks and recreation departments for information on events or organizations. Call local rehabilitation professionals and find out if there are organizations that they know about, or if they could refer you to other people with disabilities. Peers are a terrific resource to let you know what's happening or provide support.

Colleges and community centers offer classes that are a terrific way to start increasing your activity. Take a cooking class, learn a language, find out about a different culture and plan a trip. Parks and recreation programs, churches, veterans and community organizations also offer classes and programs. Get involved in local government. These could also be ways to meet people. Try something different.

Listed at the end of the chapter are sports and outdoor recreation resources. These organizations have been very successful at developing equipment and resources that support greater independence and opportunities. An example is the Association of Disabled American Golfers. They have helped create accessible carts that support mobility on a course as well as have special seating. These carts can support a person's lack of balance and limited positioning to be able to hit a golf ball. They can go into sand traps and even on the greens without damaging the course. The organization has also worked toward developing special grass that is not damaged by wheelchairs. In effect, the Association of Disabled American Golfers and others like it have opened doors that were previously shut to people with disabilities. Call them, they can get you information on equipment, events, rules, or even people in your area who are involved in that sport.

Look in bookstores under Outdoor Recreation and Sports. You can find terrific sources for ideas. Do not feel like you can only find information to help you in disabled sports resources. Each sport has a magazine promoting opportunities and equipment. You can get terrific ideas from these sources. Be creative!

The internet is also an invaluable resource. Look up information under key terms. If you want information on, say, tennis, try: tennis, wheelchair tennis, or adaptive tennis. To effectively find information, you have to approach your search from different angles.

Remember that your recreation is a very important part of your life. Get involved and have an adventure. Try something new and involve a friend. Be patient and begin by setting small goals. Have fun! Recreation is great medicine.

RESOURCES

Sports Organizations

Amputee Sports

Disabled Sports USA
451 Hungerford Drive, Suite 100
Rockville, MD 20850
(301) 217-0960
www.dsusa.org

Archery

Wheelchair Archery, USA*
c/o Wheelchair Sports, U.S.A.
3595 E. Fountain Boulevard, Suite L-1
Colorado Springs, CO 80910
(719) 574-1150

Basketball

Canadian Wheelchair Basketball Association
Suite B2-2211 Riverside Drive
Ottawa, Ontario K1 H 7X5
(613) 260-1296
www.cwba.ca

International Wheelchair Basketball Federation
5142 Ville Maria Lane
Hazelwood, MO 63042-1646
(314) 733-0933
www.iwbf.org

National Wheelchair Basketball Association*
710 Queensbury Loop
Winter Garden, FL 34787
(407) 654-4315
www.nwba.org

Billiards

National Wheelchair Poolplayer Association, Inc.
9651 Halekulni Drive
Garden Grove, CA 92841-4911
(866) 636-3371
www.nwpainc.com

Bowling

American Wheelchair Bowling Association
2912 Country Woods Lane
Palm Harbor, FL 34683-6417
(727) 734-0023
www.awba.org

Flying

Freedom's Wings International
699 S. Florida Avenue
Tarpon Springs, FL 34689
(727) 944-5756
email: president@freedomswings.org
www.freedomswings.org

International Wheelchair Aviators
P.O. Box 1126
Big Bear Lake, CA 92315
(909) 585-9663
email: IWAviators@aol.com
www.wheelchairaviators.org

Football

Universal Wheelchair Football Association
University of Cincinnati Raymond Walters College
Disability Services Office
9555 Plainfield Road
Cincinnati, OH 45236-1096
(513) 792-8625
www.rwc.uc.edu/kraimer/page1.htm

Golf

United States Golf Association Foundation Resource Center
1631 Mesa Avenue
Colorado Springs, CO 80906
(719) 471-4810, ext. 29
www.resourcecenter.usga.org

Handcycling

United States Handcycling Federation
721 N. Taft Hill Road
Fort Collins, CO 80521
(303) 670-8290
www.ushf.org

Hockey

United States Sled Hockey Association
198 Calvary Drive
Franklin, TN 37064
(615) 945-1089
www.sledhockey.org

Horseback Riding

American Competition Opportunities for Riders with Disabilities (ACORD), Inc.
5303 Falter Road
San Jose, CA 95132
(408) 261-2015

North American Riding for the Handicapped Association
P.O. Box 33150
Denver, CO 80233
(800) 369-RIDE
www.narha.org

Multisport

Casa Colina Outdoor Adventures
255 E. Bonita Avenue
Pomona, CA 91769
(909) 596-7733
www.casacolina.org

Disabled Sports USA
451 Hungerford Drive, Suite 100
Rockville, MD 20850
(301) 217-0960
www.dsusa.org

National Disability Sports Association
25 W. Independence Way
Kingston, RI 02881
(401) 792-7130
www.ndsaonline.org

Wheelchair Sports, U.S.A.
3595 E. Fountain Boulevard, Suite L-1
Colorado Springs, CO 80910
(719) 574-1150
www.wsusa.org

World T.E.A.M. Sports
2108 South Boulevard, Suite 101
Charlotte, NC 28203
(704) 370-6070
www.worldteamsports.org

Quad Sports

Bay Area Outreach & Recreation Program (BORP)
830 Bancroft Way
Berkeley, CA 94710
(510) 849-4663
www.borp.org

United States Quad Rugby Association
5861 White Cypress Drive
Lake Worth, FL 33467-6230
(561) 964-1712
www.quadrugby.com

Racquet Sports

International Tennis Federation (Wheelchair Tennis Department)
Bank Lane
Roehampton London SWI 5 5XZ
United Kingdom
(011) +44 (0)20 8878 6464
www.itftennis.com

United States Tennis Association
70 W. Red Oak Lane
White Plains, NY 10604
(914) 696-7000
www.usta.com

Recreation

National Handicap Motorcyclist Association
404 Maple Avenue
Upper Nyack, NY 10960
(914) 353-0747

National Park Service
1849 C Street, NW
Washington, DC 20240
(202) 208-6843
www.nps.gov
Golden Access Passport and information on national parks for people with disabilities.

Turning POINT (Paraplegics On Independent Nature Trips)
4144 N. Central Expressway, Suite 130
Dallas, TX 75204
(214) 827-7404

Road Racing

Wheelchair Track and Field-USA (WTFUSA)*
2351 Parkwood Road
Snellville, GA 30039
(770) 972-0763
www.wsusa.org

Shooting

National Wheelchair Shooting Federation*
102 Park Avenue
Rockledge, PA 19046
(215) 379-2359

NRA Disabled Shooting Services
11250 Waples Mill Road
Fairfax, VA 22030
(703) 267-1495
www.nrahq.org/compete/disabled.asp

Skiing

Disabled Sports USA
451 Hungerford Drive, Suite 100
Rockville, MD 20850
(301) 217-0960
www.dsusa.org

Ski For Light, Inc.
1400 Carole Lane
Green Bay, WI 54313
(920) 494-5572

US Disabled Alpine Ski Team
P.O. Box 100
Park City, UT 84060
(435) 649-9090

Softball

National Wheelchair Softball Association
1616 Todd Court
Hastings, MN 55033
(651) 437-1792
www.wheelchairsoftball.com

Table Tennis

American Wheelchair Table Tennis Association (AWTTA)*
23 Parker Street
Port Chester, NY 10573
(914) 937-3932

Track & Field

Wheelchair Track and Field-USA (WTFUSA)*
2351 Parkwood Road
Snellville, GA 30039
(770) 972-0763
www.wsusa.org

Water Sports/Recreation

Access to Sailing

6475 E. Pacific Coast Highway

Long Beach, CA 90803

(562) 437-0548

email: info@accesstosailing.org

www.accesstosailing.org

American Canoe Association

7432 Alban Station Boulevard, Suite B-232

Springfield, VA 22150

(703) 451-0141

www.acanet.org

Handicapped Scuba Association International

1104 El Prado

San Clemente, CA 92672-4637

(949) 498-4540

USRowing

201 S. Capitol Avenue, Suite 400

Indianapolis, IN 46225

(800) 314-4768; (317) 237-5656

email: members@usrowing.org

www.usrowing.org

U.S. Wheelchair Swimming, Inc.

c/o Wheelchair Sports, U.S.A.

3595 E. Fountain Boulevard, Suite L-1

Colorado Springs, CO 80910

(719) 574-1150

www.wsusa.org

Water Skiers with Disabilities Association

USA Water Ski

1251 Holy Cow Road

Polk City, FL 33868

(800) 533-2972

www.usawaterski.org

Weightlifting

United States Wheelchair Weightlifting Federation*

39 Michael Place

Levittown, PA 19057

(215) 945-1964

www.wsusa.org

Magazines

Sports 'n Spokes and *PN/Paraplegia News*

2111 E. Highland Avenue, Suite 180

Phoenix, AZ 85016-4702

(888) 888-2201

Access to Recreation

8 Sandra Court

Newbury Park, CA 91320

(800) 634-4351

*National governing body (NGB) of Wheelchair Sports, U.S.A.

Driving is an important aspect of our lives. It allows us greater independence. Many people with spinal cord injuries can relearn this skill with the assistance of a therapist with specific education in driver rehabilitation, a certified driver rehabilitation specialist (CDRS), or a qualified driver training instructor. These individuals can evaluate your need for adaptive equipment and provide the behind-the-wheel training needed to become a safe driver. Hand controls and steering devices enable people with spinal cord injuries to operate a vehicle.

HOW TO OBTAIN A LICENSE

The first step in obtaining a license is to contact your local department of motor vehicles. Each state has a slightly different procedure but most will require that you have your doctor complete a form stating that you are medically stable to drive. The form may also comment on your current medication, history of seizures, or need for adapted equipment. Even if your current license does not expire for years, you are responsible for having your driving record updated to reflect the change in your medical condition.

The next step in obtaining or updating your license is to complete an evaluation with a certified driver rehabilitation specialist or qualified driver's trainer. This person will assist you in determining the specific equipment to meet your needs and provide a "hands-on" trial of the equipment to ensure that you can resume safe driving.

Finally, if you are driving with adapted equipment, you can expect to be required to retake the driving test. Your license will be updated with the equipment restrictions. In most states, it is illegal to drive with adapted equipment that is not reflected on your license.

DRIVER TRAINING

Finding a Certified Driver Rehabilitation Specialist or Qualified Driver's Trainer

Many of the well-known driving schools are unable to offer the evaluation with specialized equipment and training that you require to resume safe driving. Many major rehabilitation medical centers and VA hospitals have driving programs for people with disabilities. The driver training instructors are usually therapists who have pursued additional training and experience to become certified as driver trainers.

If you are unable to find a qualified person who does driver training for people with disabilities in your area, contact your local department of motor vehicles, the American Automobile Association (AAA), or the Association for Driver Rehabilitation Specialists (ADED). (See the resources at the end of this chapter.)

When You Should Begin Driver Training

In the initial months after your injury, you are very busy focusing on the medical and therapeutic aspects of your rehabilitation. This is an important time to gain the skills you'll need in preparation for driving.

Driver training is usually addressed closer to discharge.

Depending on your level of skill, mobility, and transportation needs, you may want to wait at least a year or more before driving. People, especially those with quadriplegia, may make additional improvements in strength and abilities and may want to maximize their functional skills before considering driving. If changes occur in your skills, the expensive equipment and training you purchase could be no longer useful or appropriate in a few months. The decision of when to start training should be made with the guidance of your doctor and therapist. Some orthopedic or neurological restrictions and medications may affect your readiness for driving.

If your injury included a loss of consciousness, seizure, head injury, or stroke, there may be a mandatory waiting period before you resume driving. Contact your state's department of motor vehicles for details.

Training

To begin the process, you will need to complete an in-clinic assessment. Therapists will do some tests to determine your visual acuity, depth perception, spatial orientation, range of motion, balance, coordination, and reaction time. In addition, they will ask you about your previous driving experience and in what type of environment and weather conditions you would be driving in your community. This will allow the therapist and you to develop a training program to meet your specific needs.

After the in-clinic assessment, the therapist will select and educate you on the type of adaptive equipment options available and what you need. This equipment may be set up on a driving simulator to enable you to try out while the therapist is determining your ability to drive safely.

Once the appropriate equipment is determined, an in-vehicle, "behind-the-wheel" assessment is done and you will be trained in the use of the equipment. The therapist will begin teaching you to drive in a parking lot or another safe practice area. Usually the vehicle has dual control brakes for your safety. As you progress in developing your skills, you will have more complex driving opportunities and will be instructed in defensive driving techniques.

At the completion of training, you will be prepared to take the road test at your local department of motor vehicles. Often you can use the driver training vehicle, since you may not have the time or finances to already have your own vehicle modified.

EQUIPMENT OPTIONS

- *Standard hand controls.* Hand controls are mechanical levers attached to the foot pedals of the vehicle and mounted under the steering column. You push forward to brake and downward to accelerate. Hand controls eliminate the need to use foot pedals but do not interfere with others who drive with their feet.

- *Left-foot accelerator.* If only the right side of your body has loss of use, then a simple pedal can be installed to enable the left foot to do gas and braking.

- *Steering devices.* When you are using hand controls, one hand must do the gas and brake while the other steers. To make this easier, a steering device can be installed to assist in the full rotation of the wheel, making turns faster and easier.

- *Steering force reduction.* If the steering wheel requires too much force to turn or is beyond your reach, the steering box of the vehicle can be removed and rebuilt, changing the gear ratio so the force needed for turning is reduced. This includes a pump and back-up system in addition to the standard power steering.

- *Electronic dash switches.* Operation of the gearshift, ignition/start, turn signals, headlights, wipers, heater, and cruise control can be difficult if you have limited reach and hand function. Electronic switches can be installed to replace and control the dash switches and require only light pressure touch.

- *Electronic hand controls.* For people with high level quadriplegia, standard equipment may require too much effort and consequently alter your sitting balance and control of the vehicle. "High tech" computer interfaced steering and hand controls can enable a person to drive with a small diameter wheel placed close to the lap and hand controls operated in a push/pull motion against a few ounces of effort with less than 6 inches of movement.

SELECTING A VEHICLE

Your vehicle decision is based on whether you can use a car or a van with modifications. If you use a motorized wheelchair, a van equipped with a ramp entry or wheelchair lift is usually indicated. Although there are "portable" power wheelchairs available, they usually require assistance for disassembly and lifting for trunk storage. Your choice of vehicle also needs to account for who else in the family will be driving and where you will park.

If you use a manual wheelchair, you need to choose a vehicle that suits your transfer and wheelchair storage ability. Use of a rigid frame wheelchair will definitely influence how you

load it into a car and what seating is available for your passenger. The seating height of some cars may provide a level height for the wheelchair transfer to and from the driver's seat. The seating height of a truck may mean transferring up 10 or more inches, which may be difficult for some people.

What to Look for in a Car

Certain vehicles are better suited for transfers, wheelchair storage, or installation of hand controls. Your therapist can provide you with specific equipment and vehicle selection criteria. The following list offers general guidelines on purchasing an accessible car.

1. A two-door vehicle is recommended for ease of access because the doors open wider. This means that you can position the wheelchair closer for transfers and have more space for your transfer.

2. An intermediate or large car is generally recommended because the seat height may be higher and there is more legroom under the column where the hand controls are installed. Before you buy a vehicle, you should always call a vendor who installs hand controls to make sure the vehicle can be modified. Adjustable angle steering columns, air bags, and under-dash vents make hand control installation more challenging and costly.

3. Bucket seats may provide improved trunk balance and stability by providing support. However, a bench-type front seat will enable you to enter from either side of the vehicle and slide to the driver's position.

4. A center armrest/console may be desirable for long-distance driving, as well as driver stability and balance during turning maneuvers. It can also provide assistance with pressure relief when driving.

5. If you use a folding wheelchair, there should be enough room between the front and back seats to allow for storage. Also, check that seat belt anchors do not interfere with access.

6. Seat belts are required to be worn in all vehicles. In addition, seat belts and shoulder harnesses can help maintain stability and balance on stops, during turns, etc.

7. Four-wheel drive is recommended for those driving on snow and ice and is now available on many different makes and models.

8. Automatic transmission is required to operate hand controls.

9. Power steering is recommended for improved turning and to avoid over-fatiguing your arms. Most people using hand controls use the other hand to steer with a one-handed technique.

10. The steering column must be designed so the bracket for the hand controls can be attached.

11. A tilt steering column allows more space when entering and exiting and gives you wheel height adjustment.

12. Power brakes respond faster with less force of movement needed and may be required for your safety and control of the vehicle.

13. Cruise control allows the driver to maintain a steady speed without having to constantly maintain pressure on the accelerator. This helps prevent arm fatigue during long-distance driving with hand controls.

14. Power windows are recommended for drivers with limited hand function. It is also a good idea for hand-control users because it is an easier method of operation.

15. Power door locks are recommended for drivers with limited hand function or limited mobility.

16. Air conditioning is recommended for people with respiratory problems and may be considered a medical necessity for temperature regulation.

17. Remote adjustable outside mirrors give the driver optimum rear vision without having to adjust them outside the vehicle.

18. Rear window defroster and rear window wipers will improve overall vision and safety while driving.

What to Look for in a Van

The cost to buy and modify a van can be very expensive. The general guidelines for a van are similar to the car criteria. The equipment and type of van that you require will be very personalized. You must work closely with your driver training professional before making this purchase. Measurements for the wheelchair entry, headroom, and turn-around space inside the van, and whether or not you plan to transfer into the driver seat will be critical factors in your van selection. You will need to determine if a full-sized or a mini van meets your needs.

If you are not able to transfer into the driver seat, your therapist will assist you in deciding if you will need any special accommodations to your wheelchair for postural support and balance. A wheelchair is not designed to be used as the seating in a van but can be optimized to increase your safety if you cannot transfer.

What to Look for in an Installation Vendor

The vendor who will install your equipment is invaluable. They should have certifications to install specific equipment and carry liability insurance to cover the equipment and work performed.

To find a qualified vendor, ask your instructor or contact the National Mobility Equipment Dealers Association (NMEDA). (See "Additional Resources" at the end of this chapter.)

CAR INSURANCE

You will need to inform your insurance company of the change in your medical status and driving methods. They may require proof that your license has been updated with adapted equipment restrictions and that your physician feels you are medically safe to drive. Your insurance company cannot cancel your policy because of a spinal cord injury.

It is also important to tell the insurance company about any adapted equipment you have installed on your vehicle. This will ensure that it is covered under your policy.

REBATES ARE AVAILABLE TO HELP BUY EQUIPMENT

Currently, the major vehicle manufacturing companies offer cash reimbursement for adapted driving equipment. These rebates range from $500 to $1,500. General guidelines for all programs include:

1. Equipment must be installed on new/current model vehicles only.

2. Customers must have a prescription for adapted equipment written by a qualified driver trainer professional.

3. Customers receiving outside funding will be eligible for reimbursement for their out-of-pocket expenses only.

4. Programs are offered in addition to any other applicable cash rebates in effect at the time of purchase.

5. Reimbursement is intended for adapted-driving aids or conversion equipment only.

You can obtain needed forms and applications for the rebates and additional details by contacting the numbers listed below.

- Chrysler Motors Physically Challenged Resource Center (800) 255-9877
- Ford Mobility Motoring Program (800) 952-2248
- General Motors Mobility Program (800) 323-9935

THE IMPORTANCE OF TIEDOWN SYSTEMS

If you are transported by a Cabulance service, take public transportation, or even ride in your van in your wheelchair, then you need to use a tiedown system. These are the straps that secure your wheelchair to the floor of the vehicle. You should also use a pelvic and chest belt to secure you to the wheelchair. When a tiedown is secured properly, it will prevent the wheelchair from moving around. Your wheelchair brakes are not sufficient, especially in an accident.

It is your responsibility to learn how to instruct people in how to best attach the tiedowns to your specific wheelchair. Review it with your driver trainer or therapist.

Some general guidelines for use of tiedowns include:

1. Tiedown systems should be attached to the frame of the wheelchair—never secure them to removable parts such as footrests or armrests.

2. A four-point tiedown system is the safest. This system uses four straps secured at all points of the wheelchair—two in the front and two in the back.

3. In addition to securing your wheelchair, you will want to have a separate wall-mounted shoulder/lap harness. This will keep you in the wheelchair in case of a sudden stop.

4. Whenever possible, tiedowns should be positioned so that you are facing forward in the vehicle. You do not want your back lined up against a wall or window.

5. All systems should be safety tested at speeds up to 30-mph/20 G force.

HOW TO GET A DISABLED PARKING PERMIT

Contact your local department of motor vehicles for an application for a disabled person's parking permit. Most states require that your doctor sign a form indicating your need for this type of parking. Most states are beginning to issue removable placards that you can place on the dashboard or rearview mirror. Placards are more versatile than the license plates because they allow you to use disabled parking when you are in a car other than your own. If you travel, make sure that other states will honor your parking permit.

As an independent driver, you will want to know if your state has legislated a policy pertaining to gasoline stations. In many states, your disabled parking permit entitles you to purchase gas at self-service prices while having the full-service attendant dispense the gasoline. This is meant to prevent price discrimination against those who are physically unable to complete the task.

FUNDING SOURCES

Your state department of vocational rehabilitation may provide funding for evaluations, training, and vehicle modifications. Technology services and devices may be considered as a provision of the 1992 reauthorization of the Rehabilitation Act of 1973. This legislation authorizes your state to administer assistive technology services under vocational rehabilitation. To establish eligibility, you must outline your vocational objectives and the services necessary to achieve them in an individual written rehabilitation plan.

The Department of Veterans Affairs provides assistive technology equipment and related professional services to individuals who have a service-connected disability.

LOOKING TO THE FUTURE

It is your responsibility to become a safe driver and to maintain your vehicle and the adapted equipment. If you experience changes in your medical condition, have new neurologic or orthopedic problems, have increased spasticity, change your medications, or change the wheelchair you use (whether you transfer or use it as the seating in the van), you need to re-evaluate your driving.

Periodic re-evaluations may be necessary to assist you in staying safe to drive. Advances in technology have enabled people to drive a vehicle using a joystick for gas, brake, and steering. Voice control can operate the windshield wipers and turn signals, making these operations completely hands free.

Although the cost and risks involved in using such technology must be considered, people with spinal cord injuries have extensive resources and options to facilitate and prolong their ability to handle a vehicle.

RESOURCES

Organizations

American Automobile Association Traffic Safety

1000 AAA Drive

Heathrow, FL 32746-5063

(407) 444-7000

www.aaa.com

AAA's Disabled Driver Mobility Guide is particularly useful for drivers with a disability.

Association for Driver Rehabilitation Specialists (ADED)

711 Vienna Street

Ruston, LA 71270

(800) 290-2344; (318) 257-5055

www.driver-ed.org

ADED provides educational support for professionals in the field of driver education, transportation options, and equipment modifications for people with disabilities. ADED has a list of the certified driver rehabilitation specialists in your area.

National Mobility Equipment Dealers Association (NMEDA)

11211 N. Nebraska Avenue, Suite A-5

Tampa, Florida 33612

(800) 833-0427; (813) 932-8566

www.nmeda.org

This association maintains the standards of practice for manufactures and vendors of vehicles and adaptive equipment.

Rehabilitation Engineering & Assistive Technology Society of North America (RESNA)

1700 N. Moore Street, Suite 1540

Arlington, VA 22209-1903

(703) 524-6686

(703) 524-6639 TTY

www.resna.org

RESNA is an interdisciplinary association that assists people with disabilities through advancement of rehabilitation and assistive technologies. RESNA has a list of professionals who can assist you in seeking specialized information and can keep you up-to-date on research.

U.S. Department of Veterans Affairs Prosthetic and Sensory Aids Service

Mailing Code 113

Washington, DC 20420

(202) 273-8515

www.va.gov

VA reimburses the cost of equipment and installation for those veterans who are eligible for the department's services.

As an employer of an aide or attendant, you will be running a small business and will be using the skills of a personnel manager. The purpose of this chapter is to help you succeed as an employer.

DETERMINING ATTENDANT CARE NEED

The first step in looking for an attendant is deciding what activities you will need help with. This is called a "needs assessment." The checklist in table 19.A provides a general outline of duties an attendant might perform. Go through the list and mark each activity you will need assistance with. It is also helpful for you to note when and how often you need particular types of care. This will help you assess how many hours a day and how many days a week you need an attendant. If you need assistance in areas not listed, write them in the "other" spaces.

You may find you need more than one employee; for example, one in the morning and another at night if you do not need assistance during the day. Or you may need one for weekdays, then another for weekends so that each has time off. You may also want to ask someone you know to work for you when one of your regular employees is on vacation or needs time off or is sick. Sometimes previous attendants who are no longer working for you will do this, as they know your care.

CHECKLIST FOR PERSONAL CARE

Now that you have outlined your attendant needs, your next step is to clearly outline what is expected for each task listed. This may help you avoid conflicts about duties your attendant is to perform and ensure that you get the care you need. An example of a personalized care checklist is given in table 19.B. The checklist gives step-by-step instructions for one element of your personal care.

It would be impossible for you to include every detail of every step in your individualized checklist. But, on the other hand, if important information is left out, the step might not be performed properly. Here are some general guidelines for developing specific steps in an individualized checklist.

1. *Be brief.* Try to make the steps as short as possible.

2. *Put steps in correct order.* Make sure the steps are arranged in the order in which they will be performed.

3. *Include what, when, where.* Make sure the attendant knows what materials are needed and when and where the job will be performed.

4. *Avoid how.* Much of the "how to" of many steps is too detailed to include in the checklist, and you should teach them while the task is being performed. However, make sure to specify those steps that are essential or often neglected.

Items on the checklists should come from your needs assessment. It is often best to arrange the checklists in a workable order. For

TABLE 19.A. Sample Needs Assessment Work Sheet

NEED	FREQUENCY	AMOUNT OF TIME NEEDED	AM	PM
ACTIVITIES OF DAILY LIVING				
Bathing				
Dressing				
Grooming (shaving, hair care, makeup)				
Meal preparation				
Eating				
Bowel care				
Bladder care				
Turning in bed				
Transferring				
Other:				
INSTRUMENTAL ACTIVITIES OF DAILY LIVING				
Washing dishes				
Grocery shopping				
Turning on computer				
Setting up equipment				
Making bed				
Charging wheelchair batteries				
Driving van				
Errands				
Writing letters				
Answering phone				
Laundry				
Putting away items				
Housecleaning				
Child care				
Pet care				
Other:				
MEDICAL-RELATED CARE				
Pressure relief/positioning				
Medications				
Range of motion exercises				
Skin inspection				
Suctioning, respiratory care				
Other:				

TABLE 19.B. Sample Checklist for Morning Routine

GETTING READY

❑ 1. Get clothes ready.
❑ 2. Prepare bath water.
❑ 3. Check bathroom temperature.
❑ 4. Make sure needed materials are available.
❑ 5. Ensure privacy.

ROUTINE

❑ 1. Assist with bladder, such as catheterization.
❑ 2. Assist with bowel care, such as inserting suppository and digital stimulation.
❑ 3. Assist in clothing removal.
❑ 4. Move from bed to bath.
❑ 5. Wash and rinse body.
❑ 6. Assist with hair care.
❑ 7. Move from bath to dressing area.
❑ 8. Dry body thoroughly.
❑ 9. Conduct health check (such as check for pressure sores).
❑ 10. Apply lotion or powder.
❑ 11. Apply deodorant, makeup, and/or shave.
❑ 12. Assist in dressing.
❑ 13. Move to wheelchair.
❑ 14. Assist with dental care.
❑ 15. Move to breakfast area.

CLEAN UP

❑ 1. Put away all materials.
❑ 2. Clean bathroom.
❑ 3. Clean and disinfect bladder and bowel care materials.

example, if bathing is the first task to be done each morning, the bathing checklist should be first. Some people find it helpful to arrange the checklists in daily (e.g., dressing, eating), weekly (e.g., shopping), or monthly (e.g., wheelchair maintenance) order. Having the checklists arranged in an orderly manner would simplify both your and your attendant's responsibilities. The checklists then become

the basis for a very clear and complete job description for your attendant.

PREPARING A JOB DESCRIPTION

A job description needs to be very clear so that you can describe the job to a possible employee. This allows an applicant to see if the job is acceptable. Do not try to make the job sound easier or less time-consuming than it actually is in order to persuade an applicant to take the job.

The job description must be based on your specific needs and should include the following information:

- Duties and responsibilities (as described in the checklists)
- Number of hours of work per week
- Scheduled days and times
- Holiday policy
- Salary and benefits
- Qualifications, such as ability to lift a certain weight, first aid and CPR training, drivers license

If your attendant is going to live with you, your job description should include specifics about the living arrangement:

- Work hours versus leisure hours
- Days off
- Sharing of common space, including kitchen and laundry
- Roles and rights of other members of the household
- Policy on visitors
- Housekeeping
- Attendant's share of utility bills
- Acceptable behaviors (for example, smoking, drinking alcohol, partying, noise)

IDEAS FOR RECRUITING

Here are a few suggestions for finding an attendant:

- Advertise in the local newspaper
- Place flyers on bulletin boards
- Use word of mouth through family, friends, churches, and clubs
- Use an agency, either for-profit or non-profit, that will screen and refer applicants to you. This can include local Employment Security Office (unemployment benefits office).

Newspaper Ads

In writing your ad, your first objective is to attract the eyes of the prospective attendant(s). A heading of "Help Wanted" or "Handicapped Needs Help" will hardly do it. What is the attendant's incentive to help? Weekly salary? Apartment near campus? Use this as the heading to spark curiosity. Then reinforce the incentive of the heading with more detail to further develop interest.

The ad should then give a brief, but fair, idea of the obligation. Do not sugarcoat this part and you will get a more serious, mature applicant. Finally, provide a way of contacting you (first name, phone, or a purchased newspaper box number). Do not include your last name or home address for your own safety and independence.

If space and expense allow, your ad could include days of week, part-time or live-in, gender of the person with disabilities, nonsmoker if required, and time to call. Because of discrimination laws, you cannot advertise your preference of sex, age, or race. You also cannot ask for a specific height or weight, but you can require that they are able to do lifting. *(See figure 19.1.)*

FIGURE 19.1. Sample Newspaper Ad

ROOM NEAR CAMPUS IN EXCHANGE FOR WORK

Available to a quiet, reliable person able to assist a disabled woman with personal care and light housekeeping.

TWO POSITIONS AVAILABLE:
(1) Monday through Friday,
(2) Saturday and Sunday.

Two hours per day (evenings).

Nonsmoker preferred, no drugs or alcohol. References required.

WRITE TO:
P.O. BOX 123
ANYCITY, USA 00000
FOR DETAILS

Posters & Bulletin Boards

Various college campus locations, personnel bulletin boards, hospital staff lounges, and even public notice places such as those found in some supermarkets, libraries, motor vehicle offices, and community centers all offer you free recruiting places.

The strategy of content and layout for a poster or index card is much the same as for newspaper ads. Use your splashy headline to attract curiosity wherever possible, then include the newspaper ad content (see section above). With more space on a flyer, you can include more of the optional information discussed above. Reproduction costs can be minimal, and the greater freedom for attractive art forms lets you be more creative. Tear-tabs at the bottom of your flyer can be a very important feature. *(See figures 19.2 and 19.3.)*

Here are some considerations in posting your flyers:

- If you can do your posting independently, fine; if not, bring a friend with you.

- To make your message seen, pick a good place! Choose posting areas with high-pedestrian traffic of the type of people who might be interested in your offer. For instance, if you post an advertisement on a college campus, you will probably find students who are goal oriented, intelligent, and willing to learn; however, you should expect a high turnover rate due to school vacations, graduations, and transfers.

- Within these high-traffic areas, favorite places are either where people check out notices by habit (job notice board or a favorite bulletin board), or where people must wait for something and may read

from boredom (outside of elevators or cafeterias). Now that you have a good place, find a good spot within it, where your message can be seen.

- Observe any rules imposed for the posting area, and check your postings regularly to ensure no one has covered them with others.

Word of Mouth

Don't overlook the obvious: the people around you every day. Friends (e.g., from class activities or apartment living) might well include today's reserves and tomorrow's attendants. The big advantage of recruiting in this manner is your knowledge of the interested individual. Advertise during informal conversation. Family and friends may be able to identify reliable and dependable individuals who have

FIGURE 19.2. Sample Bulletin Board or Poster Flyer with tear-tabs

LIVE-IN AIDE NEEDED

Community college area
only 1 block to bus stop

Modern, 2 bedroom, 2 bath, big kitchen.
Share in return for live-in help to working
college-age man with wheelchair mobility
(2-4 hours per day, on call at night)

Mature individual preferred.
No experience necessary

Call George,
555-5555
5:30 PM to 9:00 PM for details.

To live with George, Call 555-5555

FIGURE 19.3. Sample Bulletin Board or Poster Flyer

**NURSING STUDENTS:
PRACTICE YOUR SKILLS
AND EARN MONEY**

Stable and dependable person wanted
to assist a disabled man with personal
care and light housekeeping.

Monday through Friday.
Three hours in the evening.
$8.00 per hour.

References required, prefer driver's license.

**WRITE TO:
P.O. BOX 123
ANYCITY, USA 00000
FOR DETAILS**

the ability to provide care for you—including themselves. Some people you might think least interested in working for you may pleasantly surprise you.

Using an Organization or Agency

A number of not-for-profit organizations can be sources of attendants. Centers for Independent Living assist people with disabilities to live independently and many maintain an information and referral service. So, too, do many senior centers.

Refugee employment through refugee agencies is an excellent source of help. You offer an individual exposure to advanced English, and you may have external support from the agency.

Nursing schools may be able to help you locate nursing students who want to gain experience in the skills of their future profession.

Clients of the Departments of Developmental Disabilities and Vocational Rehabilitation are another good resource. Sometimes a mentally retarded person can make a good attendant. Other people with disabilities may work out also.

You can also use a home health-care agency as a source for attendants. While they may have more training than attendants from other sources, you may not have the option of choosing your own attendant. Agencies provide insurance and other benefits to their employees, contributing to a more stable work force, but they are often more expensive to use than finding an attendant on your own.

PEOPLE WHO MAKE GOOD ATTENDANTS

There is no specific profile of the perfect attendant, but there are a few tips that may make the task of finding one a little easier:

- Consider a wide variety of options. Don't restrict yourself to someone with a specific ethnic background, culture, educational level, age, or social group.

- When selecting attendants, do not expect a long-term relationship, but do expect dependable care. Select people based on whether you feel they can be trusted. You are trying to select an employee who you believe will care for you on a regular basis.

- Family can be useful, but remember the employer/employee role. Hiring a family member may have drawbacks!

- Use friends, the SCI team, or family to help check someone out when you are really stuck or having trouble. Be careful, though, not to over-use your privilege of friendship or family ties.

- Know your own likes and dislikes. Besides basic care needs, know what you like and dislike in other people. Trust and dependable care depend on your knowing yourself and letting others know what you like. Who do you like to be around and why?

- It may be helpful to learn to assess personality (general style and behavior patterns) and emotions (how people express feelings). Pay attention to how people look, talk, and act. Notice if they are well groomed and confident. Does conversation flow smoothly?

Also, trust your gut reaction: Does it feel right to be around this person? If you feel sad, angry, confused, etc., when with this person, do you want to spend a great deal of time with them?

Another part of how you feel towards a potential attendant may be your attraction to them. Remember that you're not hiring a friend or a lover.

HOW TO HANDLE CALLS ABOUT THE JOB

Give a brief description of what the job entails: personal care, housekeeping, meal preparation, shopping, or driving. If the person is still interested, you may want to set up an appointment to meet in person or ask further questions. Here are some topics you should cover before meeting applicants:

- Do they mind doing personal care? (You may have to be specific about what this entails, such as bathing and bowel or bladder care.) Can they handle nudity that goes along with personal care? If they cannot, there is no sense wasting their time and yours. If they do not mind it, then discuss basically what is involved.

- Do not hire someone you have not seen who sounds nice on the phone.

- Describe basic household duties and other chores.

- Describe your living environment. Emphasize the positive.

- If you need a driver, find out whether they mind driving the type of vehicle you own and whether they have a good driving record.

- Discuss your social lifestyle and what you consider appropriate and allowable.

- Ask what kind of work they have done and whether they have work references.

- Ask if there are any physical or emotional limitations that would make it difficult or prevent them from doing this job.

- As if they are available to work the hours you need assistance and what flexibility they have for additional hours or filling in on short notice.

- If people call and you do not want to hire them, just tell them the position has been filled or that you are considering other people for the job.

If you get satisfactory answers and want to meet an applicant for an interview, pick a convenient time and place to meet. You may want to meet somewhere other than your home, for your own safety and independence.

INTERVIEWING

It has been the experience of many people with disabilities that half the people who make appointments for in-person interviews do not show up. Ask people to please call you if they change their minds.

Have a schedule and a job description ready for them to read. Have a notebook, to take down information like name, address, phone number, Social Security number, date of birth, ability to lift or transfer, drivers license number, social interests, and at least two work references. Other acceptable references are counselors, teachers, or ministers.

Have someone else there to write this down if you are severely disabled. This person may also prove to be a good support person during the interview.

Discuss the job in greater detail. Let the applicant know what social behavior you allow, what unexpected events may arise, the things you like doing for recreation, and what areas of your life you want to be kept confidential.

Here is a short checklist you may want to use to help discuss background:

- How many years of education have they completed?

- What kinds of work have they done and liked the best?

- Have they had any experience of being around a person with a disability?

- How long have they lived in the area?

- What are their attitudes toward disability?

- How do they deal with boredom and stress?

- Will the work hours fit into their schedule? How much flexibility do they have?

- Will they feel comfortable driving a large vehicle like a van?

- Would they mind getting up in the night to turn you or help you go to the bathroom?

- Do they understand that some physical lifting may be required?

Allow them to ask questions about your disability and lifestyle. They need to know in order to be able to do their job well. When you complete the interview, let the applicant know you will call them back with your decision. It is never a good idea to hire someone "on the spot."

CHECKING REFERENCES

As any employer would, you should not hire anyone without checking references, even if it means writing or calling out of state. A foreigner must already have a work permit and Social Security number. Unless they do, you won't be able to hire them because of FICA, federal, and state unemployment tax requirements.

When calling on references, identify yourself, explain that you are disabled and are interested in hiring one of their past employees. Describe the nature of the work they will be doing and the need for having someone dependable and honest. Tell them you would like them to tell you some things about the person. Consider asking the following questions:

- How long was the person employed?

- Was the applicant dependable?

- What about absenteeism?

- Did this person deal with money on the job?

- Do you consider this person to be honest?

- How well did the person take supervision and criticism?

- Can the person work independently?

- How was this person's rapport with other employees and supervisors?

- What was this person's reaction to stress?

- Why did this person leave the job?

- Would you rehire this person?

MAKING A CHOICE

After you have checked the references, you want to pay particular attention to the answers on dependability, honesty, working and getting along with others, why they were terminated, and their rehire status.

Are your social lifestyles compatible? Do not hire someone thinking that person will change for you or that you have the right to control that person's life. What the attendant does on off-hours should not concern you as long as it does not affect the quality of work. If you need a lot of driving done, be sure he or she has a good driving record, because it will affect both your safety and insurance.

If for any reason you do not feel comfortable with the person, do not hire that person. (See the section in this chapter on "People Who Make Good Attendants.")

Find out how long the person will be able to stay. The longer, the better—but that should not keep you from hiring the person. Some employers will hire a qualified person for a short time if they are sure they will get good service. This can be helpful when you are waiting to be discharged from a hospital. You can look for a replacement once you are home. It also helps when you need to start school or go to work.

What sort of physical and emotional health does the person have? Emotional problems can be very difficult to deal with. If you suspect but are not sure the person has emotional problems or will not be able to handle the job, hire them on a two-week trial basis.

Let the applicant know your decision within a week or less.

Finally, do not hire out of desperation. Try to remain calm and clear-headed. If you publicize as much as you can and have your schedule and job description in good order, it will increase your chances for success.

USING A LETTER OF EMPLOYMENT

To avoid any misunderstandings, it is helpful to have a written letter of employment from you to your personal assistants. That letter should cover such matters as hours of work, salary, vacation and sick leave, unacceptable social behaviors (smoking, alcohol use, profanity) and what can lead to termination, who pays when the attendant accompanies you on social outings, and the time needed for notice when the person decides to leave the job. There should also be a clear description of the arrangement made regarding taxes, Social Security, and any noncash reimbursements. The job description should be attached to the letter and referred to within it.

For live-in attendants, you should also include information about utilities (phone, newspaper, shared costs, long-distance bills) and use of your personal items such as shampoo, detergent, car, wheelchair, food, etc.

Keep a copy of the letter in your employment files.

HAVE A BACKUP PLAN

At some time or other, you will not have an attendant when you really need one. This could be due to an attendant's illness or being fired or quitting without notice. Or you may just need more than one attendant. Especially if you need care seven days a week, no one person will always be available. Personal assistants must have some days off and you need to find someone else to care for you then.

When you first get into the business of employing attendants, figure out your backup plan. You may cut down what you require, such as the housecleaning, or you can eat with a friend, or have a potluck. Do a second needs assessment and be realistic about what care you can eliminate without sacrificing your health and safety.

Arrange with a family member or friend to know your personal care, so that you can call on them to help you in an emergency. You may want to make arrangements with a neighbor (who would like to earn a little extra money occasionally) to know your care so that you can use that person when you have a need. You may make an agreement with another individual who has an attendant to share an attendant in an emergency.

Some communities have organizations that can supply attendants on an emergency basis. These may be a local visiting nurse service or an organization for individuals with disabilities. Since these resources often require advance application, assessment of needs and eligibility, and scheduling, you need to make arrangements before you are left without assistance.

Realize that the same individual doesn't have to supply all your needs. A visiting nurse will assist with bowel and bladder care, for instance, but will not perform housecleaning or run errands. You (or your family, friends, and neighbors) may know a responsible teenager who would like to earn some money performing those non-skilled tasks.

The most important part of handling the sudden loss of your attendant is planning for that situation and having several contingency plans. Remember that relatives and friends are just that...relatives and friends. If you have not overused them in the past for attendant functions, they may come through for you when you have no attendant.

WORKING WITH AND SUPERVISING AN ATTENDANT

Being a supervisor may be a new role for you. To be an effective supervisor, you need to understand the skills involved. Supervising does not mean being a boss. Supervising means working with your attendant and guiding him or her to make sure the job gets done.

This section reviews the basic skills of effective supervision. It stresses the need to work with your attendant to solve problems and to be firm when necessary. Because of the close contact between attendant and attendee, the employer/employee roles can get confused. It is important for you to use supervisory skills to stay in control, to solve problems, and to maintain a good relationship with your attendant.

REMEMBER:

Your Attendant Is Only Human

Your attendant has formally agreed to be responsible for the needs you have discussed. In return, he or she can expect your respect. He or she is a fellow human with a separate life, of which helping you is only one part. Your attendant is not bound to you for more

than the hours stated in the letter of employment. You have a perfect right to expect that services will be satisfactorily performed. At the same time, you do not have an open charge account on your attendant's time.

Do not be demanding. Use the same tact and warmth with your attendant as you would a friend. If you find you are repeatedly short-tempered toward your attendant, objectively step out of yourself for a few minutes and retrace the heated events as a third person in the room. Try to see who was really at fault or what proportions of fault were involved. Ask yourself before you confront, snap at, or argue with your attendant, "Is this a real fault of my attendant that hampers my needs, or is this a personal habit that just gets on my nerves?" If you really find your attendant is at fault, or considerably at fault, ask, when you are clearly in a receptive and unhurried mood, to "discuss something with you." Get your attendant's point of view.

If, on the other hand, you find you are mostly at fault, stop yourself. You will find that thinking before you speak helps you to maintain control. See the chapter on "Psychosocial Adjustment" for other suggestions on communication.

Expect that even an experienced attendant will forget items of your daily routine at times. Try to be tactful with your reminders.

Finally, if you need help on a special project, try to give your attendant some advance notice if possible. If it is time to change the bald tires on your wheelchair, or to do a non-routine spring cleaning of your dorm or apartment, try to let your attendant know this well in advance. This allows your attendant the courtesy of scheduling the project at a convenient time. This will help prevent the friction of a rush demand and increase the likelihood of a thorough job.

In general, show the same gratitude and respect toward your attendant as you would any other friend. Everyone appreciates a few "please" and "thank you" comments.

Confidentiality

Before you hire a person, make clear what things you want kept confidential. Respect each other's needs for privacy when using the phone, having company, or handling financial, family, and social information. Have respect for each other's bedrooms and personal property.

Remember that when you discuss personal problems with your attendant and ask for an opinion, he or she may not be able to give the best feedback or advice. You are not hiring a counselor. Many people find it uncomfortable to even listen to the problems of others, much less give advice. Do not assume that your attendant will do this. If your attendant is willing to listen to you, you should be willing to do the same when he or she needs someone to talk to.

Performance Checks

As an employer and supervisor of your attendant, it is important to provide good, clear feedback about job performance directly to your employee. For many people, "performance checks" create negative feelings such as fear, tension, or distrust. It is up to you, as an employer and supervisor, to make performance checks a positive, motivating experience. Good performance that is recognized and praised will probably make both your job (as supervisor) and your employee's job (as an attendant) much easier.

Attendants should understand that using performance checks benefits and protects them as well as you. In this model, we provide attendants with ongoing performance feedback by scheduling performance checks. Performance checks consist of the same checklist that you developed in sorting out your specific attendant care needs.

How often they should be done depends on you and your attendant. There is no rigid rule. You are responsible for giving feedback any time a job is not performed to your satisfaction. Simply remember that with a new attendant, the more often performance is checked, the sooner small problems can be solved.

As a general rule, daily duties should be checked twice monthly; weekly duties once monthly; and monthly duties every two or three months. This does not mean that you should give feedback only while doing performance checks. In addition, performance checks should not be the only time you give positive feedback when duties are performed well. When your attendant is working hard and doing a good job, a little praise goes a long way.

Deal with Conflict

Many problems arise out of making assumptions. Although a job description and letter of employment should help to clarify basic issues, rules and agreements can be broken nevertheless. Then what do you do? If there is a conflict over duties, pay, time off, social conduct, or use of property, remind the person of the agreement. If he or she refuses to comply with your wishes, act promptly and firmly to find a replacement. When you are dependent on someone for survival, it is not easy to fire that person on the spot and find another person. Allowing the situation to continue, however, will mean you will have to go without service and your health may be jeopardized.

Do not let things pile up. Deal with each issue as it arises. You may want to have an advocate help you and the attendant to settle the disagreement.

Communication

When communicating, it is not so much what you say as how you say it. Do not try to hide your feelings by saying something nice in a negative tone of voice. When talking to a person face to face, look at him or her. Evasive eye contact may convey a message that you do not want to listen to the person or deal with the issue or do not mean what you are saying. Also, communicating your appreciation on a regular basis is important so that your attendant does not feel taken for granted.

If you think your attendant is not going to listen well, consider writing letters about your concerns or put them on tape if you cannot write. Have an advocate—a friend to help settle problems or check to see if you are okay. The advocate can also follow up on your progress. Do not let something wait, especially if it relates to your care. Being assertive is very important. See the chapter on "Psychosocial Adjustment." Assertiveness is a skill that can be practiced, and several good books have been written about how to ask for what you need without being rude, nasty, or obnoxious. (See assertiveness examples below.)

ASSERTIVENESS EXAMPLES

1. A man with a disability had planned in advance to attend a concert he had long wanted to see. The day before the concert, his attendant asked him to find another driver, because the attendant had just gotten a dinner invitation from a buddy. The disabled man let the attendant know that he appreciated and understood the attendant's desire to go to dinner with the friend. Then he reminded the attendant of the previous agreement to drive him to the concert. The man also pointed out that it was too late for him to make other arrangements, so the attendant would have to fulfill the commitment to drive him to the concert.

2. A woman with a disability had hired a man to be her attendant. At the time of the interview, she explicitly stated that she had no interest in combining work with romantic involvement. After a month of employment, the man started making passes and suggestive remarks to her. She reminded him of their conversation at the time of hiring. She said she was sorry about his feelings for her, but she did not feel the same way. She stated that she would appreciate his not bringing up the issue again. If he brought it up again, she would have to let him go. The man said that he was sorry, too, and would respect her wishes. He said that he would like to give a two-week notice of termination and then leave, because he could not promise that his feelings would change.

SALARIES AND FRINGE BENEFITS

As an employer, you will be paying a salary to your employee. This money may come from different sources. Your financial resources and the community's going rate of pay will determine the amount of the salary. You may also be providing room and board and benefits in addition to salary. (See "Your Responsibilities as an Employer" sections.)

Paying Your Attendant

Many programs exist that may pay for attendant care. Each program has different eligibility criteria, application processes, and employer expectations. It is important to consider using one or more of these programs for cash wages for the attendant. It is also possible to provide noncash wages, room and board, and other benefits as the sole payment or in combination with a cash wage.

Your social worker and other health-care team members are available to explore the various options. Review the material below and then discuss your attendant plan with your social worker or others. Remember that you are the employer and (unless you use an agency) will be responsible for recruiting, hiring, firing, paying wages, and reporting cash and noncash wages for tax purposes.

Possible Payment Sources for Attendent Care

All of these programs generally require paper work such as medical documentation of need and/or financial statements. Check with each funding source about IRS and Social Security reporting requirements.

State Medicaid Programs

Contact your local program about in-home attendant care programs. Some states have special income waived programs, including funding for employed people who need ongoing attendant care after they return to work.

Workers Compensation

Each state and federal program has different requirements for funding attendant care. Ask your agency contact person for more information.

Private Insurance

Check your policy. Some policies may provide for attendant care.

Department of Veterans Affairs

VA does not directly pay for attendant care, but does supply extra pension and service-connected income to help with these expenses. Many VA medical centers provide some limited skilled nursing, and a few may also provide some unskilled help in your home. There may be funds available specifically for bowel and bladder care. Ask your nearest hospital benefits counselor or SCI center social worker for more information.

State Vocational Rehabilitation Agencies

In rare instances, a vocational program may include coverage for attendant care.

Home Health Services

Home health care is typically based on having a skilled care need, as defined by state and federal regulations. Depending on the funding source, a person may also be able to get some additional unskilled type of assistance. A physician order for skilled care is required. Home health care may be skilled nursing or therapy related, such as occupational or physical therapy. The Joint Commission on Accreditation of Health Care Organization certifies home health agencies that meet their standards; ask about certification when screening a potential agency.

Your Responsibilities as an Employer When Providing Cash Wages

If you are receiving funds with which to pay your attendant, follow the instructions from that funding source regarding:

• What payment records you must keep

• In what way and how often you will be receiving this aid

• What procedure they suggest you use in paying your attendant(s)

The source may insist on obtaining the names and Social Security numbers of each attendant to enable their direct payment. Try to persuade your funding source away from this plan. You may find that the process of a check coming "automatically" to an attendant takes away some of your natural, employer's right to bargain with an attendant. Also, whenever you change attendants, the paperwork and delay in the payroll process can result in an unearned paycheck being sent to your former attendant or a considerable delay in the first paycheck being sent to the new attendant.

Ask your funding source and local tax people whether your particular plan of funding requires any attendant you employ to declare the income on federal, state, and/or city taxes. As a matter of courtesy, inform your attendants of any taxes they must pay at the time you employ them.

Your Responsibilities as an Employer When Providing Noncash Wages

There is another way that allows you to deduct the "salary paid" from your income taxes. Quite simply, you reimburse the attendant by noncash means. As one quickly sees from the "Summary Chart of Federal Tax Forms" that follows (*table 19.C*), both the paperwork and tax costs to employee and employer are considerably less for noncash than cash wages. However, more background homework is necessary. The IRS has specific criteria regarding when and how meals and lodging can be medically deducted.

One of the simplest ways to accomplish this is to offer your attendant(s) room at your home in return for their services.

EXAMPLE: You have decided that it is best for your particular needs to hire two attendants. You rent a two-bedroom

apartment, take one bedroom for yourself, give the other to your two attendants and have the attendants split the duties. In return, you offer your attendants noncash wages in any of various combinations of room, board, electric power, and so forth.

Before deciding what item(s) to offer, you may want to explore how much of each item is currently considered medically deductible for your particular living situation. A current Revenue Ruling implies that the cost of any commodity that is offered to the attendant, beyond that which you and/or your nonattendant family would need ordinarily, might be medically deductible. For example, if you would normally need a one-bedroom apartment, but you have to rent a two-bedroom apartment for the attendant(s), then the cost difference between the one-bedroom and two-bedroom apartments might be deductible. Similarly, the cost of additional food, electric power, etc., incurred only because of the existence of the attendant(s) is possibly deductible. You may well want to limit your noncash wages to deductible items.

Choose, in priority, those noncash items that you can most easily prove you paid for by means of receipts or other records. Clearly divide these expenses objectively by the number of people in the living situation. For example, lodging and power are easier to substantiate and divide objectively than food costs.

To determine how large to make this noncash package, figure the amount of cash salary normally to be paid and equal that in noncash benefits. Whatever is NOT being offered in the noncash wage package must be understood from the beginning to be the financial responsibility of each occupant, such as food, clothing, utilities, and shaving articles. This goes for anyone who routinely shares a dwelling.

See the "Summary Chart of Tax Forms" to determine which reporting forms are still necessary. This means that you are telling the IRS who has received what amount of "income" from you. No FICA payments are required. Again, call your nearest IRS office for these forms, which will be self-explanatory.

To safeguard your own interests in case or IRS audit, see the notes at the end of the table 19.C for suggestions on your personal record keeping.

Certain filing requirements may be different from information supplied here due to such factors as personal situation of taxpayer or changing IRS policies and rulings. Use the data in table 19.C as a guideline and check your particular situation and wage method with latest policy of your nearest IRS office.

KEEPING TRACK OF ALL THIS

It is really helpful to have a file on attendants you have interviewed (acceptable and unacceptable) and also the ones you hire. You will need to keep information for tax reporting and W-2 forms. You may also want to refer to it in an emergency.

A file box is good for keeping verification forms, your copies of tax reports, and copies of canceled checks for future reference.

You could use a card file or a notebook for information on attendant applicants. The data should include:

1. Name
2. Address
3. Phone number (message number also)
4. Date of birth
5. Social Security number
6. Driver's license number
7. Date you hired them

8. Date they were terminated
9. Reason for termination

GRACEFULLY PARTING WAYS WITH AN ATTENDANT

Even though you have taken much care in screening and choosing an attendant, the one you hire may prove to be unsatisfactory. In that case, you will have to make your dissatisfaction plain and be firm in your right to expect better service. If improvement does not occur, you should move quickly to find a satisfactory replacement. An unreliable attendant is not healthy for either mind or body. You must keep control over how your own basic needs are to be met in order to meet your goal of independent living.

Try to have your attendants leave on the best possible terms, because you may want to call on them in an emergency. Also, consider developing a checklist for what needs to be completed before attendants leave. Some things to consider are:

- Make sure they have filled out a verification form (if you are receiving Chore services) before paying them.
- Make sure all basic duties are completed so the new attendant can enter a clean and orderly household.
- Get their key to the apartment/house.
- Get a forwarding address or permanent phone number. (Keep this information for your files.)

PREPARING FOR THE RECURRING CYCLE

The termination of an attendant will mean either a smooth transition into the employment of someone else or a frantic scramble for a

TABLE 19.C. A Summary Chart of Federal Tax Forms for Employers of Personal Assistance Services

IRS FORM	USED PRIMARILY TO REPORT	WHEN DUE
CASH WAGES		
W-4	Employee-desired amount of income tax to be withheld from cash wages (for "household employment" tax may be withheld only if both employer and employee voluntarily agree)	At beginning of employment. Each time employee wishes to change withholding status
SS-4	To obtain employer's identification number (EIN)	One number for employer's lifetime. For use when filing various IRS forms
942	• Cash wages of $50 or more paid to each employee in any calendar quarter • Income tax withheld during the quarter • FICA (Social Security) taxes (about 6% of each employee gross pay amount) withheld from the cash wages of any employee meeting criterion —to be matched in amount from employer (attach check for combined tax amount to FICA-942 form)	4 times a year; within 30 days of the end of each IRS-defined calendar quarter (3-month period)
940 & 580 Federal Unemployment Tax	FUTA (unemployment taxes (3.4% of first $6,000 paid to each employee) to be paid by employer; to household employees, those who paid cash wages of $1,000 or more during any calendar quarter	1/31 for wages paid in preceding year; file 940 with 580
W-2	• Cash income to employee • FICA taxes withheld from employee • Income taxes withheld (see note for W-4 form regarding household employment). Worker is responsible for paying withholding	1/31 for wages paid in preceding year or within 30 days of employee termination if before the end of year
W-3	To be filed with Copy A of W-2 and sent to Social Security Administration	1/31, with W-2

Each state has different rates. Find out your own state regulations to determine how much and how often to pay these taxes. In some states, nothing is due if wages are less than $1,000 per quarter.

NONCASH WAGES		
SS-4	Same as cash wages section.	
W-2	Value of noncash wages paid.	1/31 for wages paid in preceding year or within 30 days of employee termination if before the end of year

Notes

1. Instructions for each IRS form are usually included on the particular form. Circular E: Employer's Tax Guide is a must for employer-taxpayers. All are readily available, free of charge, from your nearest IRS office.
2. Your employees must have social security numbers; if they do not, have them file an SS-5 form with the IRS to receive one.
3. For noncash wage employers, be sure to save all bills, rent leases, payment checks, and receipts applicable to items of non-cash reimbursement. Do not attach to tax forms, but save for at least four years in case of an IRS audit.
4. For noncash wage employers, an index card statement, containing information supplied in the informal example above, has been found helpful to the personal record keeping of such taxpayers.

replacement. It depends on whether you have done your homework.

With the best planning and preparation of the new attendant, even the most experienced employer may feel insecure in the transition from old to new. Anxiety is a natural feeling for anyone moving from an established, familiar situation into one that is new or uncertain. For certain people with disabilities, this twinge of insecurity will be a little more intense due to a little more architectural—or personal care—dependency.

Studying and analyzing as many aspects of the situation as possible and then preparing for them has proven the best way to minimize that transition twinge. We hope that helpful hints of this text will best enable you to do so for yourself.

RESOURCES

Publications

Managing Personal Assistants: A Consumer Guide.

Purchase:
  PVA Distribution Center
  P.O. Box 753
  Waldorf, MD 20604-0753
  (888) 860-7244
www.pva.org

Web Sites

www.eldercare.com
CareGuide.com provides general information and housing, legal planning, assisted living, and home care resources by geographic area based on a client profile of needs that you provide. There are free quality care tools such as checklists to evaluate assisted living and nursing home facilities. This is a relatively easy site to use.

www.nfcacares.org
National Family Caregivers Association (NFCA) helps to raise awareness and support for all who provide direct care to people who are ill or have a disability.

www.senioralternatives.com
Springstreet.com offers a nationwide directory of state agencies that can help answer questions about home health care.

Making your home accessible can mean many things. Your home may need only a few changes, such as a ramp to the entrance or grab bars in the bathroom. Then again, it may need even more involved modifications, such as wider doorways and hallways, lower windows, or an elevator or lift.

As part of your rehabilitation program, your therapists may make a *home visit* with you. At that time, measurements will be taken and accessibility issues will be discussed. This will help you plan any modifications you may need. If you live outside of your SCI center's area, your therapists will still help you by using floor plans of your home and giving you printed materials as a resource.

In making your home accessible, there are many specifications to make sure any changes are safe and can meet your needs. These changes often need to be adapted to your particular situation. Your occupational and physical therapists are good resources for this information.

Your social worker can help you look at the resources you may have for designing home modifications. You will also be able to explore possible funding for this project through governmental or other community services.

This chapter makes recommendations for heights, widths, distances, and other home specifications. Before you jump into anything, let us help you figure out exactly what meets your needs. There are blank spaces by the drawings for you to fill in the requirements of your own specific needs.

Please note that throughout the chapter, we will use the following abbreviations:

inch or inches = " like 9" for 9 inches

foot or feet = ' like 2' for 2 feet

HAVE THE WORLD AT YOUR FINGERTIPS

You bring home a bag of groceries. You cruise up your ramp and into the kitchen. Placing the bag on the counter, you turn around to put something in the fridge and…Oh, no! The bag dumps over and all your oranges and apples roll to the back of the counter. Can you reach them?

Perhaps the barrier is something as simple as having a bathroom in which you need to go out in order to just turn around, or a sink that hits you right in the armpits, drenching your clothes every time you do the dishes.

It becomes apparent that most ready-made buildings were not made ready for you! So, customize them. Plan ahead and in no time your house will really be *your* home.

The diagrams of wheelchair dimensions and levels can get you started in making sure work counters, tables, doors, etc., are accessible to you and your wheelchair. *(See figures 20.1 and 20.2.)* Your therapist can help you in measuring your chair, as well as figuring out turn spaces and your reach from your chair.

FIGURE 20.1. Turning Space Required

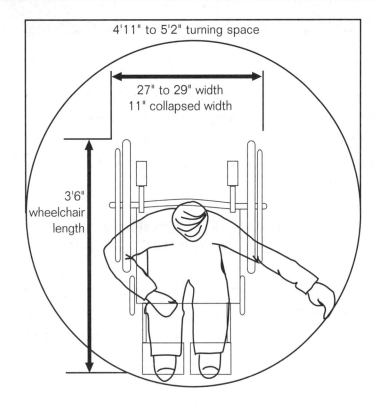

4'11" to 5'2" turning space

27" to 29" width
11" collapsed width

3'6"
wheelchair
length

Average Dimensions
Width: 27" to 29"
Length: 3' 6"
Turning space: 4'11" to 5'2"

Your Dimensions
Width: _____
Length: _____
Turning space: _____

FIGURE 20.2. Wheelchair Dimensions

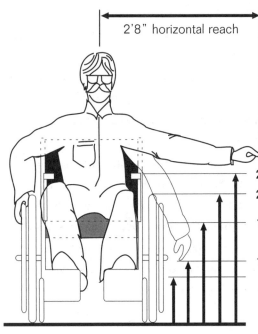

2'8" horizontal reach

Average adult reaches from a wheelchair
Vertical: 5' (4'6" to 6'6")
Horizontal working: 2'6"
Bilateral horizontal: 5'4"
Diagonal: 4'

Average Dimensions	Your Dimensions
2'5" Chair armrest level (counters, tables)	_____
2'3" Thigh level (tables, sinks, lavatories, work areas)	_____
1'8" Chair seat level (toilets, showers, baths)	_____
1'0" Downward reach (shelves, outlets)	_____
9" Foot height (toe recesses)	_____

PLANNING FOR ACCESSIBILITY

Ramps for Your House

Sometimes it seems that all the world is a staircase. Many places are wheelchair accessible because they have ramps, but others are not. The one place you should be sure has ramps, though, is your own home.

Ramps are a safe way of replacing steeper sets of stairs. Listed below are some hints on what you should consider when building ramps.

- *Length:* Safe ramp lengths should be *one foot for each inch of rise.* This means a slope of "one in twelve," 1:12, or an 8.33 percent incline. For example, if you have two 7" steps or a total 14" rise, you will need a 14' long ramp.

Exceptions to this guideline are if you have very strong arms or are using an electric wheelchair. In either of these conditions, you may be able to use a steeper ramp. We still recommend that you use the 1:12 ratio, though. You'll appreciate that when you bring home groceries or are carrying a baby in your lap!

- *Width:* The recommended width for ramps is 36" to 48". A 48" width is usually very convenient if you use marine plywood, since it comes in sheets of 4' by 8'.

- *Landings:* Landings are necessary at the top and bottom of ramps as well as at any intermediate levels where a ramp changes direction or rises more than 3". Landings at all levels should be at least 5' x 5'. *(See figure 20.3.)* The top landing should be placed so as to extend 1'6" on the latch side of the door. This means that if you want to center the platform on a 3'0" opening , a wider, 6'0" platform would be needed. If the door opens in, the platform can be 3' deep x 5' wide. *(See figure 20.3.)*

- *Railings and Edges:* Railings are best placed on both sides of the ramp, approximately 32" high and securely fastened to the ramp. They can be made of 2" x 2" or 2" x 4" lumber, or 1½" diameter pipe. The edges of the ramp should be at least 2" high to prevent wheelchair casters from going over the edge.

- *Surfaces of Ramps:* Ramps exposed to the outdoors can become extremely slippery and dangerous unless a proper nonslip surface is used. Adhesive nonskid strips, ribbed rubber matting, or a rough roofing material can be used. A broom-swept surface works well for a concrete ramp. A painted surface is not recommended as it

FIGURE 20.3. Ramps

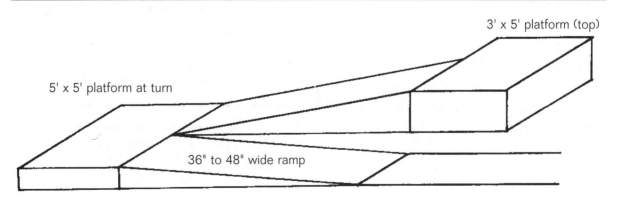

3' x 5' platform (top)

5' x 5' platform at turn

36" to 48" wide ramp

can be very slippery when wet. However, paint mixed with sand (one pound of silica sand mixed thoroughly with one gallon of paint) or a non-skid deck paint both provide nonslippery surfaces. Surfaces should not be so rough as to make wheelchair travel difficult or unpleasant.

- *Materials for Ramps:* For building a long-lasting ramp, use of treated lumber (such as plywood), concrete, or 2" x 4" slats placed crosswise is recommended. Ramps that are the means for emergency exits should be built of fire-retardant materials.

Walkways and Entrances

Walkways around your house are important to provide a solid, constant surface through rough terrain like your yard. That way, you will not have to worry about getting stuck, especially when the ground is soft due to rain or snow. That is, of course, if the walkways are built right!

Walkways should be a minimum of 42" wide to prevent slipping off the edge. To allow for wheelchair turning on corners or switchbacks, a 5' width is needed.

Entrances should have a clear, unobstructed opening of at least 32" (36" preferred) with a level or beveled threshold no more than ½" higher than the floor.

Doorways and Hallways

Have you ever gone through a doorway and mashed your fingers on the edge of a box you were carrying or smashed your fingers on your wheel because you just barely had enough room? Not too much fun, is it? So give yourself a break and plan plenty of room for your doorways.

The minimum width of doors should be 3'0" (32" clear opening). Special attachments on your wheelchair may require even wider doors. Ask your therapists to help you determine your wheelchair width. *(See figure 20.4.)*

Doorways into bathrooms or other confined spaces should swing out. Large bathrooms providing ample maneuvering space will permit the door to swing in; however, in-swinging doors are a potential hazard if you should fall and block the door. Sliding doors, pocket doors, or "break away" hardware are other alternatives.

Doors can be one of the biggest obstacles in your daily life. In fact, there are several

FIGURE 20.4. Door Width

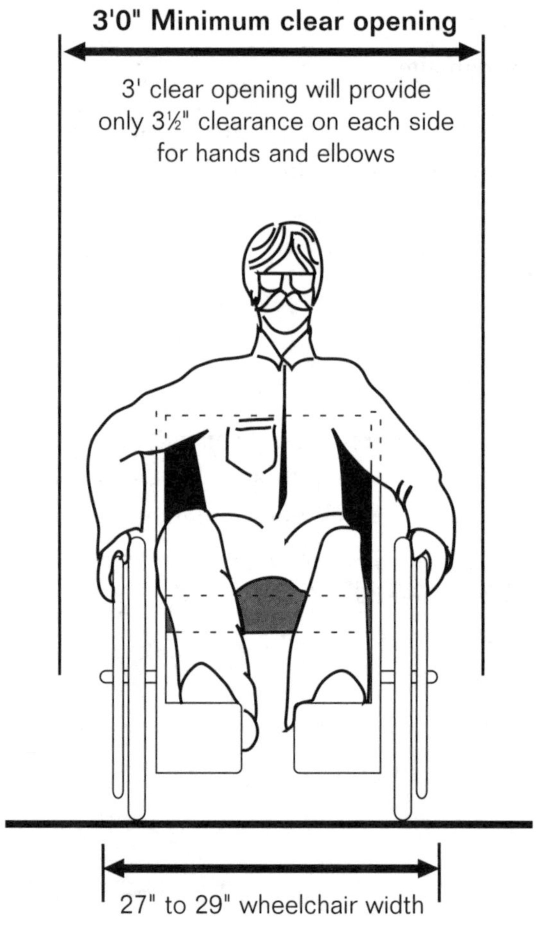

3'0" Minimum clear opening

3' clear opening will provide only 3½" clearance on each side for hands and elbows

27" to 29" wheelchair width

things about a door that you should be aware of in order to make your life easier.

1. Any door must be capable of being opened in a single motion.

2. Door latch handles are easier to grasp than round ones. Your therapist can make recommendations on various ways to adapt door handles, handles to cabinets, etc. *(See figure 20.5.)*

3. The best height for door handles is approximately 3'. Your therapist can help you evaluate your reach and determine what heights work best for you. *(See figure 20.6.)*

4. No matter how careful you try to be, the footrests of your wheelchair are going to scratch your doors from time to time. Kick plates on both sides of your doors are recommended to protect them from this kind of damage.

Hallways at least 36" wide allow wheelchair access to rooms; however, if a doorway is too narrow, turning may still be difficult. Figure 20.7 illustrates the best hallway-doorway configurations to optimize your accessibility.

Other Convenient Heights

Some modifications you may need can get lost among all the more major changes you are planning. Check out the heights and measurements given below to make sure you don't miss them:

- Counters, tables, and sinks: 27" to 33"
- Electrical outlets: 18" to 48"
- Light switch/thermostat: 36" to 42" from floor
- Wall-mounted telephones: 32" to 40" recommended; maximum height of 48"

- Closets:
  — Clothes hanger rod: maximum height of 48"
  — Shelves: maximum height of 54"
- Windows: For viewing, a low sill height is recommended (no higher than 30")

FIGURE 20.5. Latch Handle

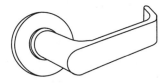

FIGURE 20.6. Door Dimensions

Door should open with single motion

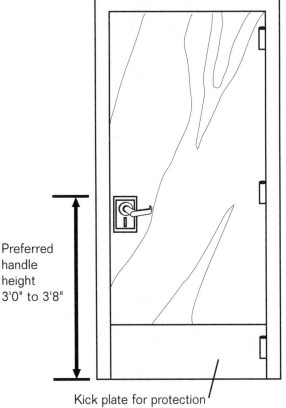

Preferred handle height 3'0" to 3'8"

Kick plate for protection from footrest

FIGURE 20.7. Hallways

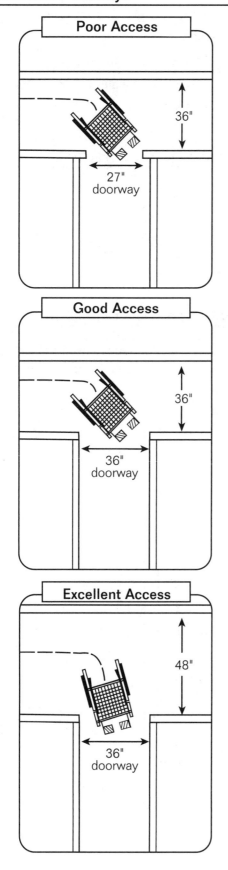

Poor Access

36"

27"
doorway

Good Access

36"

36"
doorway

Excellent Access

48"

36"
doorway

The heights of tables, beds, etc., can be easily raised using wooden blocks. Your therapists can help answer these questions for you.

Bathrooms

All bathroom fixtures and equipment must be thoroughly evaluated by you and your therapist. The height of toilet seats and the placement of grab bars are specific to you and to the type of bathroom you have.

Part of your rehabilitation process will be the evaluation of your bathroom facilities. If changes or adaptations are needed, your therapist can give you the specific details.

SAFETY CONSIDERATIONS

1. If you have to come down a very steep ramp, you may want someone to back you down the ramp to prevent you from falling out of your wheelchair.

2. Exposed hot water pipes, drain pipes, motors, and other sources of burns or abrasions should be adequately housed or insulated; preset hot water heaters to less than 120 degrees.

3. Doors to any confined space with only one exit should swing out. In-swinging doors pose a potential danger should the wheelchair user fall and block the door.

4. You may want to have two separate accessible emergency exits in case of emergency.

5. You should consider an emergency warning signal, e.g., a system to alert neighbors, fire department, police, in case of an emergency.

6. Install smoke detectors throughout your home (hallways, kitchen). If you have difficulty hearing, a system that alerts you with lights (or other means) would be a good idea.

7. Fuse boxes or circuit breakers should be accessible.

8. Provide adequate, even lighting throughout the house.

9. It is helpful to have accessible telephones near the bed and a phone jack in the bathroom; consider carrying a cordless phone with you throughout your home.

10. Have a fire extinguisher readily available and within reach.

RESOURCES

Publications

Accessible Home Design
Purchase:
    PVA Publications Distribution Center
    P.O. Box 753
    Waldorf, MD 20604-0753
    (888) 860-7244

Organizations

The Center for Universal Design
North Carolina State University
Box 8613
Raleigh, NC 27695-8613
(800) 647-6777
www.design.ncsu.edu/cud/

The Ramp Project
Metropolitan Center for Independent Living
1600 University Avenue West, Suite 16
St. Paul, MN 55104
(651) 646-8342

Trace Research & Development Center
1550 Engineering Drive
Madison, WI 53706
(608) 262-6966
(608) 263-5408 TTY
email: info@trace.wisc.edu
www.trace.wisc.edu

Web Sites

www.easyaccesshomes.com
You'll find information at Easy Access Homes on homes that are suited to the needs of your family—whether that means a home with main floor living for family members who have difficulty with stairs or a home with total wheelchair access throughout.

www.hometime.com
Hometime is an on-line source for home improvement, remodeling, and repair information. Here is where you'll find project advice and products to help you with your project.

The day of discharge may seem far away when you are first admitted to the spinal cord injury service. It will take some time for you to develop your goals for your life after discharge. With each goal, you will make decisions about where you wish to live, what you want to do, contacts you will want to make. Your family, friends, and others will be interested and involved, too. However, you are the director of your discharge plan.

PLANNING YOUR DISCHARGE

There are some important areas to consider in discharge planning. The questions listed in the forms that follow will direct your planning in these areas. Try answering these questions with your family, friends, and the rehabilitation team working with you. Every team member will be available as a resource in answering these questions. You can use this chapter as a workbook to formulate your answers to these important questions regarding your discharge. In addition, home safety and other checklist resources are available from the web sites listed at the end of this chapter.

Some people will be returning to their place of residence at the time of spinal cord injury. Others will need to make changes in their living situation. Here are a few tips to guide you when searching for the environment best suited to you.

Private Home

In addition to a home evaluation, don't forget a good safety check. A checklist is available from one of the web sites listed at the end of this chapter.

Group Living Situations

There are many types and names for shared living situations. Some options are:

- *Retirement Residence*—An apartment or single home setting that can include some physical help.
- *Assisted Living*—An apartment setting that usually includes some physical help available most of the day.
- *Adult Family Care Homes*—A small home-like setting with 24-hour caregivers. Most states require inspections and certification of these homes.
- *Nursing Home*—A skilled nursing facility with 24-hour per day RN or vocational nursing staff (LPN) who can handle complex medical problems. These facilities are regulated by state (Medicaid) and federal (Medicare) agencies.

Selecting any particular setting is a highly personal decision. The best approach is to decide what features are most important to you and find a way to check out the facility. Ask for references, have a tour, and use the checklists that follow or those from the web sites mentioned at the end of this chapter.

MEDICATIONS AND SUPPLIES

Your OT, PT, nurse, doctor, pharmacist, or prosthetics team member can answer these questions for you. For additional information, refer to the chapter on Medications.

1. What are your medication and supply needs?

    A. _____

    B. _____

    C. _____

    D. _____

    E. _____

    F. _____

2. What are the side effects of your medications?

    Medication: _____

    Side Effects: _____

    _____

    Medication: _____

    Side Effects: _____

    _____

    Medication: _____

    Side Effects: _____

    _____

Medication: _____

Side Effects: _____

_____

Medication: _____

Side Effects: _____

_____

Medication: _____

Side Effects: _____

_____

3. How and where will you get your medications and supplies refilled? (There may be a two-week lag time.)

    How: _____

    _____

    Organization: _____

    Address: _____

    _____

    Phone: _____

DESTINATION FOLLOWING DISCHARGE

Your social worker and other team members can explore the answers to the following questions with you. For additional information, check out the chapters on "Community Resources" and "Home Modifications."

1. Where will you be living?

   Street Address: _____

   City:_____ State: _____ Zip: _____ Phone: (_____) _____

2. Is your residence accessible or does it need modification?

   ❏ Accessible   ❏ Needs Modifications

   What modifications are needed?

   _____

   _____

3. How are you going to make your home and community environments barrier free?

   _____

   _____

4. How can you obtain the equipment you will need to make your home accessible?

   _____

   _____

5. Who can you contact for home modifications?

   Company or Organization: _____

   Street Address: _____

   City:_____ State: _____ Zip: _____ Phone: (_____) _____

   Company or Organization: _____

   Street Address: _____

   City:_____ State: _____ Zip: _____ Phone: (_____) _____

6. Who will pay for the adaptations?

   ❏ Individual (you personally)   ❏ Organization or government agency

   Organization: _____

   Contact Person: _____ Phone: (_____) _____

7. How will you pay for your living expenses?

   ❏ Individual (you personally)   ❏ Organization or government agency

   Organization: _____

   Contact Person: _____ Phone: (_____) _____

FOLLOW-UP AFTER DISCHARGE

Your social worker and the rehabilitation team will explore the answers to these questions with you. For additional information, refer to the chapter on "Community Resources."

1. What contact will you have with the medical center or another hospital after discharge?

   _____

   _____

2. How will you get appointments and who will pay for them?

   ❑ Individual (you personally)   ❑ Organization or government agency

   Organization: _____

   Contact Person: _____ Phone: (____) _____

3. Will outreach staff from local community agencies visit you after discharge? ❑ Yes   ❑ No

   If so, who? _____

4. If you need help with your daily routine, who will be available?

   Organization: _____

   Contact Person: _____ Phone: (____) _____

   Organization: _____

   Contact Person: _____ Phone: (____) _____

5. What community agencies will provide services after discharge?

   Organization: _____

   Contact Person: _____ Phone: (____) _____

   Organization: _____

   Contact Person: _____ Phone: (____) _____

6. How will you travel home?

   _____

7. Who will pay for and arrange your travel plans?

   ❑ Individual (you personally)   ❑ Organization or government agency

   Organization: _____

   Contact Person: _____ Phone: (____) _____

8. Do you know whom to call if you have a problem at home?

   Name: _____ Phone: (____) _____

FAMILY, ATTENDANT, AND CAREGIVER EDUCATION

Your OT, nurse, social worker, or other team member can help answer these questions. For additional information, refer to the chapters on "Attendant/Management," "Bowel Management," and "Skin Care."

1. What is your care routine? _____

_____

_____

2. How much help will you need? _____

_____

How long do these tasks take to perform? _____

When do these tasks have to be done? _____

_____

3. Who will pay for attendant services?

❑ Individual (you personally)   ❑ Organization or government agency

Organization: _____

Contact Person: _____ Phone: (____) _____

4. If you need an attendant, how will you find that person?

_____

_____

5. How and when does the attendant training begin?

_____

_____

6. Can you train someone else in your care routine?   ❑ Yes ❑ No

If so, how are you going to do it? _____

If not, who can do it for you?

Organization: _____

Contact Person: _____ Phone: (____) _____

7. How will the spinal cord injury unit or other rehabilitation staff be involved with the training?

_____

_____

8. Who can you contact if you have a crisis with your attendant?

Name: _____ Phone: (____) _____

Name: _____ Phone: (____) _____

THOUGHTS ABOUT DISCHARGE

Your rehabilitation team, peers on the SCI unit or in the community, and others can help answer these questions. For more information, refer to the chapters on "Psychosocial Adjustment" and "Sexuality."

1. How can you be sure that you are ready to be discharged?

_____

_____

2. Are your family members, friends, and/or attendant ready for your discharge?

_____

_____

3. Have you thought about the questions others may ask you about your injury or your wheelchair? What will you say?

_____

_____

4. What will you do about your feelings once you are home?

_____

_____

5. Will you talk with your family or friends? Do you want to meet other individuals who are disabled?

_____

_____

6. Support group?

Organization: _____

Contact Person: _____ Phone: (_____) _____

7. Peer Counseling?

Organization: _____

Contact Person: _____ Phone: (_____) _____

8. Individual counseling?

Organization: _____

Contact Person: _____ Phone: (_____) _____

TRAVEL AND TRANSPORTATION SERVICES

Your PT, OT, or social worker can be your resource. For more information, refer to the chapters on "Community Resources," "Driver's Training," and "Recreation."

1. Do you have accessible public transportation in your area?

   ❑ Yes (list organizations and phone numbers below for easy reference)   ❑ No

   Organization: _____ Phone: (___) _____

   Organization: _____ Phone: (___) _____

   Organization: _____ Phone: (___) _____

   Organization: _____ Phone: (___) _____

   Organization: _____ Phone: (___) _____

   If no, how will you get around? _____

   Who can you call for assistance? _____

   Name: _____ Phone: (___) _____

   Name: _____ Phone: (___) _____

2. What do you need to know about accessible public transportation?

   _____

   _____

3. What about driving? Will you be the driver or will you need someone to drive for you?

   _____

4. How do you get a valid driver's license?

   _____

   _____

5. How will you pay for transportation?

   ❑ Individual (you personally)   ❑ Organization or government agency

   Organization: _____

   Contact Person: _____ Phone: (___) _____

EQUIPMENT

Your PT, OT, and prosthetics team members will work out the answers to these questions with you. For more information, refer to the chapter on "Equipment."

1. If you need adaptive equipment, how and where will you get it?

   Organization: _____

   Contact Person: _____ Phone: (_____) _____

   Organization: _____

   Contact Person: _____ Phone: (_____) _____

2. Who pays for the equipment?

   ❑ Individual (you personally)   ❑ Organization or government agency

   Organization: _____

   Contact Person: _____ Phone: (_____) _____

3. How do you get the equipment repaired or replaced?

   Organization: _____

   Contact Person: _____ Phone: (_____) _____

   Organization: _____

   Contact Person: _____ Phone: (_____) _____

ADDITIONAL RESOURCES FOR VETERANS

For more information, see the "Community Resources" chapter.

PVA representative:

   Name: _____ Phone: (_____) _____

SCI Coordinator for the VA medical center closest to you:

   Name: _____ Phone: (_____) _____

Veterans Benefits counselor:

   Name: _____ Phone: (_____) _____

HOME AT LAST

The entire team can be a resource in answering these questions. For more information, check out the chapters on "Vocational Rehabilitation," "Recreation," "Attendant Management," and "Psychosocial Adjustment."

1. In addition to your personal care, what will you do all day?

_____

_____

2. What kinds of vocational training, employment, or volunteer opportunities are you interested in?

_____

_____

Where can you find assistance to help you get started in those areas you listed?

Organization: _____

Contact Person: _____ Phone: (____) _____

Organization: _____

Contact Person: _____ Phone: (____) _____

3. What will you do for fun and relaxation?

_____

_____

Where can you find assistance to help you get started in those areas you listed?

Organization: _____

Contact Person: _____ Phone: (____) _____

Organization: _____

Contact Person: _____ Phone: (____) _____

4. What will you do if a crisis occurs (for example, if your wheelchair breaks down or your attendant quits)?

_____

_____

5. What is your financial situation?

_____

_____

RESOURCES

Web Site

www.senioralternatives.com/dynahtml/sla/ rrcheck.html

A retirement residence checklist and other resources are available.

www.agenet.com

A retirement residence checklist, nursing home checklist, assisted living checklist, home safety checklist, and other resources are available.

www.hcfa.gov/medicare/nurshm1.htm

An informative guide to choosing a nursing home is available.

Pain After Spinal Cord Injury

Pain is common after spinal cord injury (SCI). As many as 40 percent of individuals with SCI report pain that is severe enough to interfere with their daily activities. All SCI patients will experience some pain at some time in their life, though in many this is temporary and mild.

KINDS OF PAIN

There are several different kinds of pain after SCI. A person with SCI usually has one kind of severe pain but may have two kinds of pain at the same time. The different kinds of pain can be described by location and by duration.

Location of Pain

Muscle, Bone, or Tendon Pain

This kind of pain often results from injury to muscles, bones, or tendons that might occur from overuse, overstretching, or falls. Such pain can last for weeks or months if your body reacts to the injury with inflammation or muscle spasm. Common sites for this pain are shoulder, low back, neck, and hands, but other sites may show this pain as well. This pain often feels like aching, grinding, or gnawing; it is often worse with activity but relieved by rest. Technical names for this kind of pain and its causes include myofascial pain, heterotopic ossification (bone formation in soft tissues), arthritis, and shoulder impingement.

Nerve Pain

Pressure, irritation, or stretching to a nerve can cause pain. This can occur at the neck or back where the nerves exit the spine, such as

with a slipped disk. Nerves may also be compressed at the elbow or at the wrist causing pain; one type of wrist pain due to nerve compression is carpal tunnel syndrome. This nerve pain can feel like aching, heaviness, tingling, or numbness in the fingers or hand.

Spinal Cord Pain

This is a mysterious kind of pain. Cutting the spinal cord does not cause immediate pain, but SCI can, over days to weeks, lead to pain. This kind of pain that originates in the spinal cord or brain is often called central pain or neuropathic pain. It may be felt at the level of the spinal cord injury as a band around the body—this band may be hypersensitive to touch or may tingle or burn. Another type of central pain is a burning, tingling, or freezing sensation below the level of the injury—this may be felt in the feet or around the anus. Another type of central pain is a brief shock or jolt or a series of quick shocks, often in the legs. This spinal cord pain can develop days to weeks after a spinal cord injury or it can develop years later if there is additional damage to the spinal cord—for example, if an expanding fluid-filled cyst develops in the spinal cord (called a syrinx or syringomyelia). Those with incomplete SCI or with cauda equina injuries (low level SCI at Ll or lower) often have the most severe spinal cord pain, though even those with complete SCI may experience this pain.

Internal Organ Pain

Your internal organs, such as your stomach, intestines, or bladder, develop pain if they are overstretched. Thus, if you have constipation and your intestine overstretches or if your bladder overfills, then you will feel internal abdominal pain. Internal organs may also develop pain if they lose their blood flow; for example, a heart attack causes chest pain when blood flow is interrupted to the heart. Internal organ pain (also called visceral pain) may be difficult to distinguish from spinal cord injury pain. If pain suddenly worsens, it is important to identify new internal organ pain and distinguish it from a worsening spinal cord problem or from a new muscle, bone, tendon pain. Bladder overfilling, constipation, inflammation of the gallbladder, and heart attack are medical emergencies that require prompt treatment. After spinal cord injury in the neck (cervical) or upper back (thoracic at T6 or higher), sensation from the heart, stomach, intestines, and bladder may be dulled and difficult to pinpoint but it is not usually absent.

Headache Pain of Autonomic Dysreflexia

People with SCI above a T6 level can develop autonomic dysreflexia, where blood pressure rises rapidly to high levels in response to bladder overdistension or some other pain stimulus below the SCI. Blood pressure may rise to dangerously high levels (i.e., greater than 180 mm Hg) making this a medical emergency. See the chapter on "Autonomic Dysreflexia". Such high blood pressures often cause headache. This is a kind of pain unique to spinal cord injury.

Duration of Pain

Acute or Short-Duration Pain

Sudden onset, severe pain is worrisome since it may indicate a medical emergency (for example, autonomic dysreflexia, heart attack, bleeding ulcer, or appendicitis); get prompt medical advice or go to an emergency room. Mild to moderate pain lasting days to weeks is often muscle, bone, or tendon pain. It will usually resolve on its own and can benefit from treatment with rest and mild pain medications.

Chronic or Long-Duration Pain

Long-duration, severe pain lasting months to years with a burning, tingling, shock-like, or shooting quality is often spinal cord pain. Long-duration, mild to moderate pain that is aching in quality and that is aggravated by activity is usually muscle, bone, or tendon pain; occasionally, this muscle, bone, tendon pain can be severe.

DIAGNOSIS

Diagnosis is identifying the cause of a patient's kind of pain or pains. To diagnose pain, a doctor listens to your symptoms, examines you, may obtain blood and urine tests, may take X-rays or other imaging studies, and may order electrical tests of your nerve and muscle (EMG). If the cause of the pain can be identified, then treatment can be targeted against that kind of pain. Sometimes the cause of the pain cannot be definitely identified. Then treatments are undertaken on a trial-and-error basis.

TREATMENT

Muscle, Bone, or Tendon Pain

Muscle, bone, and tendon pain can often be improved or cured. Treatments include short-term rest (less than 3 days), cold or heat, stretching, massage, mild analgesics (e.g., acetaminophen), anti-inflammatory medications (e.g., aspirin, ibuprofen). Other treatments for persisting pain may include improving posture, modifying mobility techniques, injections into muscle or joint, and electrical stimulation to skin (TENS or transcutaneous electrical nerve stimulation).

Nerve Pain

Nerve pain may be improved by avoiding pressure or stretching, e.g., a wrist splint can relieve night pain due to carpal tunnel syndrome or an elbow pad may relieve pain due to pressure on the ulnar nerve. Splints, pads, alternate wheelchair armrests, positioning aids for computer use, a neck collar, and TENS may help. Occasionally surgery can help relieve pressure on nerves and thus relieve pain. Medications that have been used for this nerve pain include antidepressants, antiseizure medications, mild pain medications (such as acetaminophen, aspirin, ibuprofen) and strong pain medications (such as oxycodone and methadone).

Spinal Cord Pain

This spinal cord pain is often not fully relieved by current treatment. Various treatments can lessen the pain. Stretching, active exercise, electrical stimulation of the skin, relaxation exercises can help.

Certain medications can lessen this spinal cord pain: antidepressants such as amitriptyline and desipramine and antiseizure medications such as carbamazepine (Tegretol®) and gabapentin (Neurontin®). Topical pain medications (such as capsaicin or analgesic balm) may also help. At times, narcotic medications are used, such as codeine and methadone. Disadvantages to narcotics are that they cause constipation and some tolerance to the pain relief develops.

Various surgeries have been tried to relieve this spinal cord pain, but none with consistent success; these include cutting pain pathways in the spinal cord and implanting an electrical stimulator to interrupt the flow of pain signals to the brain.

Expanding vocational, social, and recreational activities may help distract you from the pain. Sometimes other factors such as depression or muscle, bone, joint pain or visceral pain can add to spinal cord pain; by treating these other factors, the spinal cord pain will be less. Other treatments exist such as herbal medicine, chiropractic manipulation, and acupuncture, but their effectiveness in spinal cord pain has not been demonstrated.

WHAT SHOULD YOU DO, IF YOU HAVE PAIN?

- *New Severe Pain, No Clear Cause*: Seek medical advice promptly. If you experience associated shortness of breath, light-headedness, dizziness, sweating, or passing out then consider ambulance transport to an emergency room. If there is associated high blood pressure, then seek treatment for autonomic dysreflexia (see Chapter 11).

- *New Muscle, Bone or Tendon Pain:* Apply cold for 15 minutes, take acetaminophen, rest for 3 days. Seek medical advice if there is no improvement after 5 days.

- *New Mild to Moderate Pain, No Clear Cause:* If you have any constipation that might be aggravating pain, then treat as needed. If you have any new loss of sensation or new weakness, then seek medical advice promptly. Try acetaminophen with or without ibuprofen (avoid ibuprofen if you have a history of stomach ulcer, kidney disease, or allergy to ibuprofen or aspirin) and rest for 3 days; if there is no improvement or there is worsening then seek medical advice.

- *Long-Standing Pain, No Clear Cause:* Try daily gentle stretching. Try acetaminophen with or without ibuprofen (avoid ibuprofen if you have a history of stomach ulcer, kidney disease, or allergy to ibuprofen or aspirin). Try a hot water bottle. (Use only warm water; do not use very hot water that will cause burns on skin with poor sensation. Do not use a heating pad on skin with poor sensation.) Seek medical advice if pain persists and it interferes with sleep or daily activities.

WHAT IS SUBSTANCE ABUSE?

Substance abuse is a major social and health-care problem that affects millions of people. It is a problem that cannot be denied when considering spinal cord injury (SCI). Substance abuse is known to be a major factor in the cause of many traumatic injuries. People who abuse substances are at a higher risk for physical complications and poor adjustment following SCI. For many people with SCI, substance abuse is a short-term solution to the challenges of disability that creates long-term problems.

What is substance abuse? Substance abuse refers to the harmful use of alcohol and a variety of other drugs that affect mood and thinking. These drugs include prescription medications as well as illegal drugs. The prescription medications most commonly abused by patients are those used for the treatment of pain (e.g., "narcotics" such as morphine, oxycodone, codeine, Tylenol #3®, or Percocet®), spasticity (e.g., Valium®), anxiety (e.g., Xanax® or Ativan®), or sleep. Illegal drugs include cocaine, heroin, and a variety of other chemicals that have no accepted therapeutic value. Marijuana is a more controversial drug in terms of its usefulness with problems such as spasticity versus its use to alter mood. Regardless of the intended purpose, the excessive or inappropriate use of any of these substances can have serious consequences for the person with SCI.

Alcohol or drug use is a factor in at least 50 percent of the incidents that resulted in SCI.

Almost half of all people with SCI use prescription medications with abuse potential; among these people, almost 25 percent admit misusing medications on one or more occasions.

Substance abuse problems that exist prior to an SCI tend to continue or worsen.

SUBSTANCE ABUSE AND YOUR REHABILITATION

SCI is a catastrophic event in the lives of all patients and their families. Your life has been disrupted and changed in many ways. Rehabilitation and adjustment are difficult and demand that you put out significant effort and learn new skills. It can be frightening and exhausting and seem like more than you can handle. Unfortunately, alcohol and drugs offer many people a quick escape from the demands of rehabilitation.

The realities of SCI can be very harsh. Because of this, it is very important that you understand that the relief provided through alcohol and drugs is, at best, temporary. There is no problem faced by people with SCI that is so difficult that it can't be made worse by the additional problem of substance abuse.

For some people, substance abuse after SCI is simply a return to their lifestyle before injury. If drugs or alcohol played a role in your injury, you are at high risk for returning to your old habits and patterns. Problems with substance abuse tend to continue and worsen after SCI. Perhaps you think of yourself as "cured" or believe you've "learned a lesson." That's great. Many people change after life-threatening experiences.

But to keep up the progress, you need to recognize that the temptations will be plentiful. Alcohol and drug use may be common among your friends and family. There may be pressure to fit back in and act just the same as before your injury. You will need a plan for dealing with social situations where others are using drugs or alcohol. Talk with your healthcare providers about strategies or programs where you can find support for your good intentions.

For other people, substance abuse after SCI is more subtle. Perhaps you never had a problem with alcohol or never used drugs for recreation. You may have never wanted to "get high." How can you be at risk for substance abuse?

Unfortunately, many of the same medications that have legitimate medical uses in SCI also have potential for misuse. Many people develop problems with increasing doses of prescription medications for pain, anxiety, or sleep. Work closely with your doctor to develop a rational plan for using these types of medications. Be particularly aware that drinking alcohol while using these types of medications is dangerous.

It is well known that the excessive use of alcohol, prescription medications, or illegal drugs is particularly harmful to the person with an SCI. Physical complications such as skin ulcers, urinary tract infections, malnutrition, and constipation are more common among people who abuse substances. Psychological complications such as depression, lack of motivation, and poor concentration are common in people with SCI who have such problems.

Adjusting to SCI will require all of your attention, skills, and abilities. You can't afford to burden yourself with another problem, even

if it seems like you feel better in the short term. Alcohol and the common prescription medications are actually central nervous system depressants. They slow down your body and your thinking and will eventually make problems like depression worse.

DO YOU HAVE A PROBLEM?

The professional journals are full of complicated criteria and different tests for determining whether or not an individual has a problem with substance abuse. A simple but useful tool is the CAGE. The CAGE questionnaire is often used in medical settings to screen for problems with alcohol. It has been adapted to include drugs (both prescription and illegal).

- Have you ever attempted to **C**ut down on drinking or drug use?
- Have you ever felt **A**nnoyed with criticisms about your drinking or drug use?
- Have you ever felt **G**uilt about your drinking or drug use?
- Have you ever used alcohol or other drugs as an **E**ye-opener?

Answering yes to any two of these questions has been shown to be predictive of alcoholism or substance abuse. If your answers suggest you might have a problem but you disagree, you might want to consider another way of thinking. John de Miranda (1992) said that the important question to answer is, "Does a person's alcohol or drug use create negative consequences?" These problems can occur in any area of a person's life: personal relationships, work, recreation, finances, and physical health and wellness. Stated another way, **if your drug or alcohol use causes you any problems, then you have a substance abuse problem.**

WHAT TO DO

Many resources are available to people who might have a substance abuse problem. This chapter lists some references that contain valuable information. You can ask your health-care provider to refer you to professionals for a more complete evaluation to determine how best to help you.

There are many different ways to find and get help with a substance abuse problem. **But it all begins with you**. Only you can take an honest look at yourself and your behavior. Only you can make the decision to change the way you drink or use prescription medications. Think about it. It might be one of the most important decisions you will ever make as you continue in your rehabilitation.

RESOURCES

Books and Pamphlets

Inform Yourself: Alcohol, Drugs, and Spinal Cord Injury. J. de Miranda.

Purchase:
> Novation, Inc.
> 2165 Bunker Hill Drive
> San Mateo, CA 94402
> (415) 578-8047

Alcohol, Drug, and Prescription Medicine Use after SCI

Purchase:
> Medical College of Wisconsin
> SCI Center
> 5000 West National Avenue
> Milwaukee, WI 53295
> (414) 259-2785
> www.mcw.edu

Web Sites

www.caas.brown.edu

The Center for Alcohol and Addiction Studies at Brown University offers training, research, and medical resources.

www.health.org

National Clearinghouse for Alcohol and Drug Information (NCADI) is the information service of the Center for Substance Abuse Prevention of the Substance Abuse and Mental Health Services Administration. NCADI is the world's largest resource for current information and materials concerning substance abuse.

Hardly a day goes by that we don't hear or read something about the many benefits of regular exercise. The physical and psychological benefits of leading a fit and healthy lifestyle are well documented and widely publicized. Now that you have a spinal cord injury, it is even more critical that exercise becomes an integral part of your life. During your rehabilitation immediately following your injury, you will be exercising regularly under the guidance of skilled health professionals. Once you are discharged from the hospital, keeping exercise as a part of your daily routine is essential to maximize your abilities and overall health.

TYPES OF EXERCISE

There are several types of exercise that are important aspects of a well-balanced program targeted to improve fitness and function. They are:

- *Muscular strength and endurance training.* Strengthening enhances the ability of muscles to contract with maximal force. Endurance training increases a muscle's ability to contract repeatedly and to resist fatigue.

- *Cardiorespiratory or "aerobic" conditioning.* Aerobic conditioning improves the body's ability to use oxygen by training the heart and lungs to work more efficiently during a sustained activity.

- *Stretching.* Flexibility exercises help to maintain or increase the length and mobility of muscles to allow the body to move as normally as possible.

Stretching is addressed in detail in the chapter on "Range of Motion." Therefore, the goal of this chapter is to discuss recommendations for muscular strength and endurance training and aerobic conditioning when you have a spinal cord injury.

BENEFITS OF EXERCISE

Exercise to improve muscular strength and endurance is important for a number of reasons:

- Allowing you to get from point A to point B whether you push a manual wheelchair, drive a power wheelchair with your hand or head, or have the ability to walk.
- Enabling you to move and take care of yourself as independently as possible.
- Protecting yourself from injuries.
- Supporting good upright posture.

Exercise to improve aerobic fitness is important for the following reasons:

- Improving your heart and lung function both during rest and during activity.
- Improving blood flow and oxygen delivery to muscles and skin.
- Decreasing the risk of heart disease.
- Improving the body's ability to burn fat.
- Providing the body with more energy for daily activities.

Exercise in terms of general health also helps in many ways:

- Keeping your bones strong.
- Maintaining an ideal body weight.
- Improving control of blood sugar.

- Allowing you to participate in leisure and recreational activities you enjoy.
- Sleeping well.
- Feeling good about yourself and your body.

MUSCULAR STRENGTH AND ENDURANCE TRAINING

Depending on your level and classification of spinal cord injury, you will have some muscles that are within your voluntary control and some that are not. See the chapter on "SCI Anatomy and Physiology." The muscles above your level of injury should not be neurologically impaired, but following your SCI they may be weak due to prolonged bedrest or inactivity. If you have a complete or sensory incomplete/motor complete injury, the muscles below your level of injury no longer work and thus they cannot be strengthened. If you have a motor incomplete SCI, some of the muscles below your level of injury work, but they are significantly weaker than normal. The goal of strengthening exercises is to encourage the muscles that you can voluntarily control to work as well as possible.

During your rehabilitation hospitalization, your physical and occupational therapists will design an exercise program to target all muscle groups that need training. Each program is tailored specifically for each person, depending on the level and extent of the spinal cord injury. For example, people who cannot move anything but their heads and necks will have a program to target the neck and breathing muscles, while people who have the ability to move all of their limbs will have extensive programs to target all muscle groups.

Whether you are completing your initial rehabilitation or have had your spinal cord injury for a while, the general recommendations for strength training are as follows:

- Address all muscle groups.
- Start with a low load and work up gradually.
- The load should allow you to complete all repetitions of the first set of 8 without struggling.
- Complete 2-3 sets of 8-12 repetitions.
- Rest for at least 1 minute between sets.
- Once you can do 3 sets of 12 easily, progress that exercise by one of the following:
  — increasing the resistance,
  — decreasing the rest between sets, or
  — adding more strengthening exercises for that muscle group.

For endurance training of a muscle or muscle group, the above recommendations apply with the following differences:

- Use a lighter resistance that allows you to complete 15-20 repetitions easily.
- Do 3-5 sets of 20-30 repetitions.
- Limit the rest between sets to less than 1 minute.

What Is Functional Exercise?

Often the best exercises are those that are "functional" or mimic the activities that you need to do in your everyday life. Your occupational and physical therapists encourage this type of exercise because it helps you learn to coordinate your movements while improving muscle strength and endurance. One example of a functional exercise is using your finger so move small objects from one place to another, which helps to improve the use of your hand muscles for self-care activities. Another example of a functional exercise is practicing your transfers over and over using the appropriate technique so that your shoulder muscles become well trained to move your body weight. All of the skills you practice in therapy sessions have a purpose; if you are not sure why you are doing a particular exercise or activity, ask your therapist to explain.

Functional exercise is also doing all the activities that you need to do each day to take care of yourself and move around. Managing your legs for dressing, driving or pushing your wheelchair, transferring, and writing are examples of everyday activities that help to keep your muscles working well.

CARDIORESPIRATORY OR AEROBIC CONDITIONING

When you hear "aerobic exercise" you may think of jogging, cycling, aerobic dance class, or other exercise activities you did before your spinal cord injury. Now that you have a spinal cord injury, you need to consider other ways to improve your cardiorespiratory system through aerobic training. Depending on your level of injury, you will have different options available to you. Some ideas are:

- Pushing a manual wheelchair
- Seated aerobics videos
- Arm ergometry
- Handcycling
- Seated rowing
- Wheelchair road racing
- Swimming
- Seated cross-country skiing
- Adaptive sports (basketball, quad rugby, tennis, etc.)

The goal of aerobic type training is to get your heart and lungs working harder than they do during your everyday activities. With consideration of SCI, the American College of Sports Medicine recommends the following for effective aerobic conditioning:

- Intensity (how hard): 50–80% of peak heart rate
- Frequency (how often): 3–5 days per week
- Duration (how long): 20–60 minutes per exercise session

How to Measure Heart Rate

When you are participating in an aerobic exercise program, it is important to monitor your heart rate (or pulse). If you cannot take your heart rate yourself, teach someone to do it for you. Here is how you check your heart rate:

1. Use a watch or clock that counts seconds.
2. Find your pulse with your first two fingers (not your thumb) at one of two places:
   (a) on the thumb side of your wrist with your palm up, just above the fold of your wrist
   (b) at one side of the middle of your neck, right next to your windpipe
3. Count the number of beats that you feel in a 10 second period.
4. Multiple the number of beats times 6 to get your heart rate in beats per minute.

   Example: 20 beats felt in 10 seconds
   20 x 6 = 120 beats per minute, which is the heart rate

Peak Heart Rate and Training Zones

In the above recommendations for cardiorespiratory training, you see that aerobic exercise requires that you work at 50–80% of peak heart rate. What does this mean? Peak heart rate is defined as:

220 minus your age.

So for a 40-year-old person, this is how to calculate appropriate intensity of exercise.

$$220 - 40 = 180,$$

which is the peak heart rate

50% of 180 = 90 beats per minute
(.5 x 180 = 90)

80% of 180 = 144 beats per minute
(.8 x 180 = 144)

So the training heart rate zone for a 40-year-old person would be between 90 and 144 beats per minute.

Rate of Perceived Exertion (RPE)

Another way to determine the intensity of exercise is to judge how hard the exercise feels and compare it to a scale. The rate of perceived exertion (RPE) scale is illustrated in Figure 24.1.

When you are working in an aerobic training zone to improve fitness, you should be exercising between level 4 "somewhat strong" and level 7 "very strong." If the exercise feels "moderate," you need to work harder; if it feels more than "very strong," you need to slow down. Research has shown a good correlation between heart rate training zones and the RPE.

FIGURE 24.1 Rate of Perceived Exertion

0	Nothing at all
0.5	Very, very weak
1	Very weak
2	Weak
3	Moderate
4	Somewhat strong
5	Strong
6	
7	Very strong
8	
9	
10	Very, very strong
	Maximal

Borg Scale (from Borg, A.A.: Med. Sci. Sports Exerc., 14:377, 1982)

When to Use RPE Instead of Heart Rate to Gauge Exercise Intensity

If your spinal cord injury is at or above T6, the part of your nervous system that controls heart rate is impaired. When you exercise, your pulse does not increase the way it should, so it is difficult to get to an actual training zone based on heart rate response. Instead, it would be better to use the RPE scale and base the intensity of the exercise on how hard you feel you are working. The RPE scale can also be reliably used for injuries below T4 and is often a more convenient way to measure how hard you are working, especially if it is difficult to stop the exercise to take your pulse.

The Importance of Warm Up and Cool Down

You should not ask your body to start or stop an intense exercise abruptly. In order to allow the muscles, joints, and cardiovascular system to warm up and cool down properly, you should perform at least 5 minutes of low intensity exercise before progressing into your training zone and after completing a work out. Gentle stretching during the warm up and cool down periods also helps to prevent injury.

BASIC EXERCISE PHYSIOLOGY PRINCIPLES

The following are some general exercise concepts that you should know for muscular strength and endurance training as well as aerobic conditioning. The principles are important whether you have a new SCI or have been injured for a long time and are starting a new exercise program. These exercise "rules" apply not only to people with a disability but to anyone expecting body changes through exercise.

- *Overload principle:* You must exercise at an intensity that is greater than your everyday activities in order for your body to get the physiologic benefits of that exercise. The intensity of the exercise must also be progressively increased over time so that the exercise continues to be challenging. The frequency (how often), the intensity (how much), and the duration (how long) can be modified to make a given exercise a more challenging one. A general recommendation is to increase the intensity of an exercise approximately every 2 weeks.

- *Specificity principle:* Your body reacts to an exercise based on what that exercise is intended to do, with little carry over for other training goals. For example, lifting weights increases strength, but has little effect on cardiovascular fitness. Additionally, the best way to train for an activity is to actually do that activity. For example, if you want to improve your swimming time, you should swim a lot!

- *Reversibility principle:* Have you ever heard the phrase, "Use it or lose it"? Basically, the positive effects from exercise remain as long as you continue and progress in your exercise program. As soon as you stop exercising, your body will get weaker and lose all the hard work you've put into it. (And you lose fitness much quicker than it took to gain it!) So it's important to remain committed to your exercise program so you don't have to start over from scratch.

CRITICAL CONSIDERATIONS WHEN EXERCISING WITH AN SCI

- *Skin protection:* Don't forget to do your pressure releases. Avoid staying in one position for a long time that could compromise your skin.

- *Bone density:* People with long-standing spinal cord injury tend to have osteoporosis, which weakens your bones. Be careful not to drop heavy weights on yourself and avoid falling during exercise activities.

- *Temperature regulation:* Remember that your body's ability to regulate temperature may be impaired by your spinal cord injury. Be especially cautious when exercising in very warm or very cold environments. Dress appropriately in layers that can be added or removed and use a spray bottle of water to cool yourself when needed.

- *Hydration:* Be sure to drink plenty of water before, during, and after exercise. Balance your water intake with bladder management.

- *Bladder and bowel:* Empty your bladder or leg bag just before exercise and maintain a consistent bowel maintenance program to avoid autonomic dysreflexia and accidents during exercise.

- *Body stabilization and hand supports:* If your trunk muscles are paralyzed, you may need to use special straps or belts to stabilize your body while you exercise. If your hand strength is impaired, you may need to use special gloves, elastic wraps, or Velcro cuffs to secure your hands to equipment.

- *Illness:* If you are sick, take a break from your exercise program until you are feeling better.

- *Low blood pressure:* If your resting blood pressure is less than 80/50, you should wear an abdominal binder and compressive stockings while exercising. Blood pressure often drops in people with SCI when exercising, so know the symptoms of hypotension and monitor how you are feeling while you exercise.

- *High blood pressure:* Be aware that some types of exercise may induce autonomic dysreflexia for some people with SCI above T6. Know those symptoms, discontinue exercise if they arise, and seek medical attention as appropriate.

- *Pain*: Discontinue exercises that aggravate pain.

Medications Can Affect Exercise Tolerance

It is not uncommon to take many medications to manage spinal cord injury issues and other medical conditions. Some medications directly affect the body's tolerance for and reaction to exercise. Be sure to check with your doctor about the medications you take and ask specifically if there are special considerations for any of your medications in relation to exercise.

A FEW FINAL SUGGESTIONS

- Try to choose exercise activities that you like. You are far more likely to continue a program that is fun. Consider exercising with a friend or family member to keep things enjoyable.

- Avoid overdoing it. The phrase "no pain, no gain" means that you should work hard; it does NOT mean that you should work to the point of hurting yourself. You may get some minor muscle soreness as you begin or progress an exercise program. This discomfort should resolve within a few days.

- Fitness and function are much more important than "looks." Your goal should not be

to have big bulging muscles like a body builder, but rather to have a healthy and fit body that allows you to do what you need to do without fatigue and pain.

- Good nutrition is a very important aspect of your exercise training program. Refer to the chapter on "Nutrition" and contact your dietitian if you have specific questions.

- Ask for help. If you are unsure how to do a particular exercise or need guidance for starting a new exercise program, ask your SCI therapists to get you going in the right direction.

Regardless of your level of injury, exercise is important to keep your body as physically fit as possible. You need your muscles to be strong, your heart to be healthy, and your body to be flexible to maximize your independence. Make a commitment to yourself to keep exercise a part of your healthy lifestyle!

RESOURCES

Sources for discussion and advertisement of adaptive exercise equipment, seated exercise videos, and disabled sports, exercise, and recreation can be found at the websites of the following magazines and organizations.

Web Sites

www.palaestra.com
Palaestra is a forum of support, physical education, and recreation for people with disabilities.

The purpose of this chapter is to give you information about alternative kinds of medicine practices. In a general sense, alternative medical practices are those that are not usually practiced in hospitals by your conventional doctor or taught in medical schools. Some examples include herbal supplements, chiropractic manipulation, massage, and acupuncture.

Public interest in alternative (or complementary or integrative) medicine is increasing. One large survey estimated that one out of every three adults in the United States used some type of alternative medicine. Over 70% of these adults, however, did not feel comfortable telling their doctor about this. Another study showed that one out of every four people taking prescription medicines also took some kind of herbal "natural" supplement. A natural supplement can be an herbal, mineral, botanical (phytomedicine, from plants), vitamin, or nutraceutical (chemically derived) substance.

Most people think that natural supplements cannot do any harm. Unfortunately, some of these preparations can have negative side effects or interfere with the way your prescription medication is supposed to work. It is very important that you ask your doctor before taking any natural supplement, especially if you are already taking a prescription medicine. It is also important to talk to your doctor before trying an alternative therapy, such as acupuncture or chiropractic manipulation. Some types of chiropractic manipulation can alter the stability of your spine (see section on "Potential for Harm").

DIFFERENT CATEGORIES OF ALTERNATIVE MEDICINE

- *Phytomedicines:* The use of plants and plant products as therapeutic agents and supplements. This includes herbs, minerals, vitamins, and botanical sources.

- *Nutraceuticals:* Supplements that are advertised as "natural" but are derived from chemicals instead of plants and are not prescription drugs regulated by the Food and Drug Administration.

- *Energy Medicine:* A variety of therapies that focus on altering "energy fields" in the body and thus affecting metabolic and functional processes. This includes acupuncture and homeopathy.

- *Nutritional Medicine:* The use of nutritional interventions to treat chronic and acute diseases, prevent illness, and maintain health.

- *Mind/Body Medicine:* The use of techniques from a variety of cultural and belief systems to identify and treat disorders thought to be influenced by a mind and body connection. This includes counseling, prayer, meditation, and visualization.

- *Physical and Manual Medicine:* This term encompasses several different fields such as massage, chiropractic, rolfing, reiki, and therapeutic touch.

RESEARCH ON ALTERNATIVE MEDICINES

Until recently, it has been difficult for doctors to gain access to reliable information. Some doctors are interested in learning more about alternative medicines, and some are not. Most physicians and scientists agree that there is not enough research about most alternative medicine treatments to support prescribing these treatments.

Alternative medicine is not taught in conventional medical schools, where your physicians were trained. Also, many more physicians prescribe alternative therapies in Europe than in the United States. The obstacles to incorporating alternative medicines into mainstream health care include lack of research proving effectiveness, economics, ignorance about treatments, and lack of standards of practice.

In 1993, Congress established the Office of Alternative Medicine within the National Institutes of Health (NIH). The purpose was to determine the effectiveness of alternative medical treatments and help with integrating treatments found to be effective into mainstream medical practice. In 1998, this office became a free-standing entity called the National Center for Complementary and Alternative Medicine.

It is very important to discuss any alternative treatments you are considering with your doctor, so that you and your doctor can determine safety and effectiveness for your individual situation.

NATURAL SUPPLEMENTS ARE NOT FDA REGULATED

Prescription and over-the-counter (not requiring a prescription) medicines have been approved for safety and effectiveness by the Food and Drug Administration (FDA), an agency of the federal government. To be approved, each medicine must go through a very costly and lengthy process of research. The FDA determines what the active ingredi-

ents are, the effectiveness of the ingredients, safety, possible side effects, contraindications, and the recommended doses.

The FDA does not approve or regulate any natural supplement, for several reasons. Herbal and botanical preparations contain multiple ingredients. The quantity, quality, and strength of these ingredients are often unknown and can vary from plant to plant. These compounds are not patentable, so the herbal manufacturer could never make enough money to afford to seek research trials and approval from the FDA.

The federal government is concerned, however, about the growing number of people who take natural supplements. In 1994 Congress passed the Dietary Supplement Health and Education Act to establish an Office of Dietary Supplements, governed by the NIH. This agency has begun collecting and compiling scientific information and research about the safety and effectiveness of dietary supplements. The web site is dietary-supplements.info.nih.gov.

DISTRIBUTION

In the United States, herbs are sold as nutritional supplements. Herbs can be taken in many forms: infusions, concoctions, potions, salves, oils, compresses, and pills. Until recently, these supplements were found only in health food stores, but now they are found in most pharmacies and supermarkets and are marketed over the internet.

In addition, herbal supplements are being added to food and drink products sold in grocery stores. It is possible to find St. John's wort added to cereal and ginseng or ginkgo biloba added to drinks. Product research is not available to determine the potency of herbs added to food or possible food/herb interactions. Nothing on food labels describes potential interactions of herbs with prescription medicines.

EFFECTIVENESS

There is limited evidence, based on scientific research, that some categories of alternative medicine are effective. Several studies have indicated that therapeutic touch, massage, and acupuncture have improved both acute and chronic medical conditions. Some natural supplements have shown promising improvements in particular diseases and their symptoms.

There is still a lot of research that needs to be done. Despite the lack of scientific evidence, many people who use alternative medicine have a very strong belief system that the particular modality works for them, based on their own individual experience.

POTENTIAL FOR HARM

Although there is still a great deal we do not understand about these treatments, we do know that some harmful results and side effects can occur. Always read the labels of any natural supplement, since there are several on the market that contain trace amounts of toxic substances (such as arsenic).

Never take a natural supplement if you are also on a prescription medicine without first consulting with your doctor. Herbs can either enhance or destroy the actions of other herbs or drugs. St. John's wort, for example, should not be taken at the same time as prescription antidepressants because it can cause toxicity. Ginkgo decreases platelet function and can greatly increase the effect of aspirin or coumadin, beyond the therapeutic range into a potentially dangerous range. Two published reports link ginkgo with bleeding from the eye

and in the brain (subdural hematoma). Guarana contains more caffeine than many cups of coffee. People with high blood pressure should avoid guarana, goldenseal, ma huang, and licorice.

Some people believe that because a substance is "natural," it can do them no harm. This is not the case. Rattlesnake venom, strychnine, and a large number of plants, for example, are "natural" substances that are also highly toxic.

SOME CONTRAINDICATIONS

Here are some alternative therapies and contraindications for them—that is, some conditions that would indicate against the use of a particular alternative therapy. This list by no means covers all the areas of alternative medicine. Tables 25.1 and 25.2 list the adverse effects of some nutritional supplements and herbs. Herbs can enhance or block the action of other drugs. Many SCI patients have "polypharmacy" ("many drugs"), with a long list of prescription drugs. Herbal preparations that may affect endocrine function and neurogenic bowel and bladder should be used with extreme caution. Tables 25.1 and 25.2 are only examples of some of the preparations more commonly used by people with SCI and are by no means comprehensive lists. In people with SCI, herbals may cause gastrointestinal distress or anticholinergic effects (resulting in urinary retention or constipation), which may trigger autonomic dysreflexia (AD). Those subject to AD should avoid products that increase blood pressure, such as ephedra, guarana, goldenseal, ma huang, and licorice. Many products can potentiate (make more potent) the effects of aspirin or coumadin. Some products, such as guarana or echinacea,

TABLE 25.1. Adverse Effects of Selected Nutritional Supplements

SUBSTANCE	USE	ADVERSE EFFECTS
Calcium	Bone strength	Can cause constipation in high doses
Omega III Fatty acid	Hypertension and Arthritis	Trouble breathing; allergy to seafood, nausea, bloating, skin rash
Folic Acid	Deficiency	Reduces effectiveness of bactrim and dilantin
Glucosamine	Arthritis	Fatigue, headache, upset stomach, diarrhea, heartburn, constipation, loss of appetite
Iron	Anemia	Can cause constipation, and increase risk of colon cancer in high doses
Melatonin	Insomnia	Do not take with thyroid medications
Potassium	Deficiency	High doses can cause fatal cardiac arrythmias
Selenium	Nutrition	Metallic taste in mouth, darkened nails, dizzy spells, nausea
Vitamin A	Antioxidant	Can cause headaches, itching, and liver toxicity in large doses
Zinc	Healing	Toxic in large doses, causing nausea, diarrhea, vomiting, abdominal pain

may cause a diuretic effect, causing dehydration, tachycardia, orthostatis, and impaction.

- *Acupuncture* should not be used over open wounds or soft-tissue infections. Use with caution in skin that does not have normal sensation. Placement of acupuncture pins can increase spasticity.

- *Chiropractic therapy* should not be used if there is any possibility of spinal instability, recent surgery, neurological changes, or presence of spinal cord syrinx. People with spinal cord injury are more at risk for osteoporosis below the level of injury, and osteoporotic bones are more prone to fracture. Forceful chiropractic maneuvers can cause shearing of skin that lacks sensation and cause skin wounds. See your SCI doctor before considering any chiropractic treatment.

- *Native American sweat lodges* should generally not be used by people with spinal cord injury, since excessive sweating causes dehydration. Dehydration can cause severe constipation and bowel impaction and lead to urinary tract infections and decubitus ulcers.

HEALTH PLAN COVERAGE

The majority of insurance plans offer limited coverage for nutrition counseling, biofeedback, psychotherapy, acupuncture, preventive medicine, and chiropractic and osteopathic medicine. You should check with your healthcare plan before starting any new treatment.

TABLE 25.2. Adverse Effects Associated with Selected Herbs

SUBSTANCE	USE	ADVERSE EFFECT
Echinacea	Immune boost	Toxicity with steroid drugs, tincture form may contain alcohol
Feverfew	Headache	Mouth ulcers and swelling, loss of taste, anticoagulant effect*
Garlic	Hypertension	Anticoagulant effect*, low blood pressure, increased effect of anti-diabetic drugs
Ginkgo biloba	Memory	Anticoagulant effect*
Ginseng	Multiple	High blood pressure, insomnia, rapid pulse, asthma, anticoagulant effect*
Guarana	Stimulant	Insomnia, anxiety, irritability, dehydration, rapid pulse, headache, tremors, heartburn
Hawthorn	Cardiac	Low blood pressure, fatigue, nausea, sweating
Kava kava	Pain	Do not take with alcohol, may enhance drugs like valium, dry skin, red eyes
Licorice	Multiple	Swelling, high blood pressure, lowers potassium levels
St. John's wort	Depression	Photosensitivity, enhances caffeine effects, toxic levels of antidepressant medicines
Saw palmetto	Prostate	Can alter tests for prostate cancer, can interfere with iron absorption
Valerian	Anxiety	Blurred vision, headache, nausea, enhances effects of alcohol and drugs like valium

*anticoagulant effect: Your body produces natural chemicals that will clot your blood (coagulate) if you start to bleed. Your doctor may prescribe a medicine that decreases your body's ability to clot blood (anticoagulant medications or "blood thinners"), to protect you from diseases such as a stroke or heart attack. Medications such as aspirin, heparin, and coumadin are anticoagulant medications. If you take a "natural" substance that enhances the anticoagulant effect of these medications, you could bleed too easily.

RESOURCES

Publications

The Complete German Commission E Monographs: Therapeutic Guide to Herbal Medicines. M. Blumental. American Botanical Council, 1998.

Professional's Handbook of Complementary and Alternative Medicines. C. Fetrow. Springhouse, 1998.

Fundamentals of Complementary and Alternative Medicine. M. Micozzi. Churchill Livingstone, 1996.

PDR for Herbal Medicines. N. Montvale. Medical Economics Company, 1998.

The Medical Advisor, the Complete Guide to Alternative and Conventional Treatments. Time-Life Books, 1996.

Natural Medicines. J. Jellings. Pharmacist's Letter.

Web Sites

www.altmedicine.com
Alternative Health News Online provides alternative, complementary, and preventive health news.

nccam.nih.gov
The National Center for Complementary and Alternative Medicine at the National Institutes of Health conducts and supports basic and applied research and training and disseminates information on complementary and alternative medicine to practitioners and the public.

www.HealthAtoZ.com
HealthAtoZ is a comprehensive health and medical resources developed by healthcare professionals and includes web sites, interactive tools, community tools, and information centers.

dietary-supplements.info.nih.gov
This web site provides information about the Office of Dietary Supplements, including its origins, programs, activities, and scientific resources. It is organized to help you quickly and easily find the information you seek.

Each person is unique and may require different types of equipment. Keep these things in mind when considering your equipment needs. Equipment can:

- Increase your independence
- Protect you against injury
- Protect your skin
- Provide postural support and prevent deformity
- Help prevent injury to a caregiver
- Improve your comfort
- Have high maintenance needs

Frequently, people see equipment and think it would be perfect for them. But once they buy it, they find out it does not do for them what they thought it would. Into a closet it goes. To prevent this from happening, consult your medical team. Ask if the particular item is useful with your injury. Whenever possible, try the equipment out first. Your therapist may be able to help set this up.

There are a few things that equipment should not do. It should not:

- Make life more difficult or complicated
- Be detrimental to you or your caregiver
- Increase the clutter in your home
- Break the bank

To ensure safety, avoid costly repairs, and extend the life of your equipment, it is important to perform routine maintenance care. Refer to your instruction manuals for proper care and function of all equipment. You are responsible for maintenance of your equipment. You can either do it yourself, have a caregiver assist you, or use a local medical equipment supplier. Before repair or maintenance is needed, identify someone in your community who can assist you. It is important to identify a supplier that is familiar with your specific equipment. This will expedite maintenance and repairs in the future.

Funding for equipment will vary between individuals. Depending on your insurance or care provider, there may be no assistance for the cost of the equipment or it may be covered completely. If necessary, your healthcare provider can help write a medical justification for needed equipment. Most funding sources require equipment to be medically necessary. Funding for replacement equipment also varies.

Another variable between spinal cord injury facilities is the procedure for equipment ordering. Responsibility varies from facility to facility as to which discipline evaluates and orders equipment and as to how to obtain replacement equipment after your discharge. Learn the appropriate procedure to receive the fastest service. Plan ahead. Delivery can take several weeks.

A tremendous amount of medical equipment is advertised. Selecting the correct equipment can be confusing. Purchasing the wrong equipment can be costly. Your rehabilitation staff members have been trained to evaluate and recommend the equipment that will best fit your specific needs.

This chapter discusses some categories of equipment and general purpose of the equipment. Some general use reminders are also given.

WHEELCHAIRS

Many types of wheelchairs exist. A wheelchair can be for everyday use or only for sports. You or someone else can push manual wheelchairs. You can push them with your arms or feet or a combination of both. A power wheelchair moves by a motor that you or someone else can control, by hand movements, head movements, or breath control. It is important to match the type of wheelchair you get with:

• Your type of injury

• Your skill level

• Your home environment and community needs

• Your postural needs

• Your means of transportation

• Your skin protection needs

It is very important to get the right size wheelchair for your body. A poorly fitting wheelchair can contribute to shoulder, neck, and arm pain. There are many factors to consider. It is very important to have your therapist work with you to determine the best wheelchair for you. Whenever possible try out the chair you are selecting. Be sure the chair you are trying is set up like the one you will order so your test ride will be more accurate. You wouldn't buy a new car without trying it out, would you?

Your wheelchair is your mobility. If you do not take care of your wheelchair you may be stranded somewhere when it breaks down. A few things to remember:

• Keep your wheelchair clean

• Keep the bearings clean

• Be sure the wheel locks are adjusted correctly

• Be sure the tires have the recommended air pressure

• Keep all nuts and bolts tight

• If you use a power wheelchair, be sure to maintain the batteries as recommended

CUSHIONS AND POSITIONING EQUIPMENT

People with SCI often do not have their back and stomach muscles working to help them maintain correct posture. Positioning equipment helps maintain posture. Positioning equipment is anything that is used to help maintain your body in a certain position. It can be used in bed or in a wheelchair. It can be used just to position one part of your body or the whole thing. A wheelchair cushion is a specific type of positioning equipment meant to pad your bottom when you sit. All positioning equipment should:

• Protect your skin

• Help maintain correct postural alignment

• Be comfortable

Positioning devices and cushions can be as basic as foam. Some cushions use air, gel, molded foam, or a combination of these. Others can be custom molded to fit you exactly. Most people do not need these.

Many people think that pressure mapping alone (a device that measures where you put most of your weight on the cushion) will tell them what cushion to use. This is not true. What is best for you depends on many factors:

• Pressure mapping results

• How much postural support you need

• Your skill level

• Your skin protection needs

• Your ability to care for the cushion (some are more complicated than others)

HOSPITAL BEDS AND MATTRESSES

Hospital beds can be used to increase independence. They can also provide caregivers with improved ease of care and personal safety. Hospital beds are available in fully electric or semi-electric styles. Wheels can be removed at home to make the bed the same height as the wheelchair. A wide variety of mattresses are available. It is very important that the mattress match your needs in regards to protection of skin, comfort, and ease of mobility. If you change your mattress it is important to check your skin more thoroughly the first few days for any increased pressure areas. Consult your medical team to assess the best bed and mattress to suit your needs.

Bed rails and trapezes are available. Trapezes can cause injury if used incorrectly.

BATHROOM SAFETY EQUIPMENT

There is a wide variety of bathroom safety equipment currently on the market. This equipment should be determined for your use based on your ability, skin protection needs, and body size. The size and layout of your bathroom will also factor into the equipment recommended. One example is a bathtub transfer bench. The bench extends over the side of the bathtub to make transfers easier and safer. Other examples include raised toilet seats, grab bars, and hand-held showers.

It is important to check equipment regularly for cracks in the surface and framework. Falls and injuries to the skin can occur if you use damaged or unsafe bathroom equipment. Grab bars should be installed securely following the manufacturer's recommendation.

TRANSFER EQUIPMENT

Mechanical Lifts

Lifts are available for use with dependent transfers to increase your safety and the safety of your caregivers. Lifts work well for transferring to and from the bed, wheelchair, and shower/commode chairs. Some lifts allow transfers off of the floor.

Lifts can be electric or hydraulic. Most can accommodate weight up to 600 pounds. They are relatively easy to use, but can be dangerous if used incorrectly, used with the wrong sling, or broken.

A variety of slings are available. It is strongly recommended to use a sling that is easily removed. DO NOT sit or lie on the sling for any length of time as it might cause skin breakdown.

Be sure to get training for safe use of lifts.

Transfer Boards

Transfer boards bridge the distance between one surface and another to increase safety and improve independence. The type of transfer board will depend on your size and ability. Many shapes, sizes, and lengths are available.

Check equipment regularly. If your transfer board is cracked, replace it to decrease the risk of falls or injury. *REMEMBER:* When using a transfer board ALWAYS LIFT your bottom. Sliding can cause skin breakdown.

EQUIPMENT FOR SELF CARE

Adaptive equipment is used to increase and improve independence and safety while performing self-care. There are devices for feeding, food preparation, dressing, bathing, grooming, toileting, and communication. For example, reachers, which come in many varieties and lengths, are used as an extension of your arm to access items from your wheelchair. A dressing stick can make it easier to put on or remove clothing.

Sometimes you only need an adaptive device during early rehabilitation. Once your muscle strength is improved or you learn special techniques, the device may not be necessary. For instance, an adapted spoon may be necessary at first to feed yourself. Some people learn to weave the spoon handle between their fingers. They no longer need to use an adapted utensil. Other times the use of an adaptive device is the only way a task can be accomplished with little or no assistance.

People have different opinions about the use of adaptive equipment. Some people do not like to use equipment. Others don't mind. It's your choice. A piece of equipment gathering dust on the shelf is a waste of money and space. Your therapist can help you to decide what equipment will be most useful.

UPPER AND LOWER EXTREMITY SPLINTS AND BRACES

Splints are prescribed to prevent or correct deformity, prevent joint stiffness, and decrease pain. Splints and braces can substitute for weak or absent muscle strength. They increase function and safety. They may be made of metal or molded plastic. They may be simple or complex with many moving parts. Splints and braces must fit correctly to be useful. Learn how yours should fit so that the splint or brace functions correctly and your skin is protected.

Your therapist will instruct you in the correct wearing schedule and precautions to protect your skin and joints. Be sure to look at your skin at least twice a day for pressure areas. If you notice a red spot that does not fade within 20 minutes, stop wearing the splint or brace and notify your therapist. You should also notify your therapist if you have swelling or pain.

AMBULATION DEVICES

Many different devices exist to help people walk more easily, including canes, crutches, and walkers. Specialized shoes and shoe inserts can also be used. Using special shoes or a cane can correct your walking pattern. Correcting your walking pattern can

- Increase your safety
- Increase the distance you are able to walk
- Increase your walking speed
- Decrease pain
- Prevent future muscle and joint problems

Because deviations in walking are very subtle, it is important to have a trained professional help determine what will help you best. Even if you have gained new strength in your legs and can now "safely" walk without your crutches, you should check with your healthcare provider before throwing them away. There may be another reason for you to use them. The ambulation device may be helping to protect your back and hips from problems years down the road.

Remember to monitor your ambulation device and specialized shoes for uneven wear or cracks. These can lead to falls. Use your ambulation device as directed to avoid falls and to protect your joints.

EXERCISE EQUIPMENT

Individuals with SCI may have special needs regarding exercise. Your therapist will assist you in establishing a home exercise program that will meet your needs. Be aware of any restrictions or limitations due to your spinal cord injury. Exercise equipment supplements your home exercise program and can increase or maintain function.

It is not necessary for you to turn your home into an exercise gym. A lot of expensive equipment is purchased with great intentions and ends up not being used. A few small pieces of equipment can be recommend by your therapist that will ensure a successful home exercise program without taking up a lot of space or costing you a lot of money. Adaptive equipment is available for individuals with limited upper or lower extremity function.

DRIVER TRAINING AND ADAPTIVE EQUIPMENT

Technology has made it possible for people with very little muscle strength to be safe and independent drivers of motor vehicles. Many factors must be considered when selecting a wheelchair and vehicle combination. It is recommended that you work with an expert in this field to ensure the vehicle and wheelchair are compatible with the modifications that are necessary for your independence and safety. For information see the chapter on "Driver Training."

COMPUTER ACCESS

The use of computers and the availability of adapted access to computers have mushroomed over the past several years. General use computers routinely come with software that makes access easy to modify.

A computer can change the life of its user. A thorough understanding of the user's abilities and goals is important before purchase of a computer and software. An assessment will determine factors such as how much memory is necessary, how mobile the computer must be, what input devices are needed, and how the output is to be received.

ENVIRONMENTAL CONTROL UNITS

An environmental control device is anything that assists people with manipulating functions in their environment, such as the heating and cooling system, lights, and other electronic appliances. It can be as simple as a garage door opener or as complex as a multitask, voice-activated environmental control unit.

People with SCI, especially those with high level quadriplegia, may be unable to activate environmental control functions in their work, home, and school environments in the usual way. They may be unable to open and close the door, turn on and off the light, operate the thermostat, or answer the phone.

Sometimes a person is able to perform all but a few activities. In this case it may be possible to modify just those devices. For instance, if the person has mobility but not strength in the upper extremities and is unable to pick up the phone receiver, a speakerphone can be used. One-item controllers such as X-10 modules are readily available and reasonably inexpensive. These allow the user to operate the device from a remote switch the way the remote control on the television works.

An environmental control unit (ECU) is a battery or AC powered device that can make it possible for people with extensive disabilities to independently perform tasks they would otherwise be unable to perform. It enables the user to manage several electronic functions through a single device. An added benefit to an ECU is that it can provide peace of mind through the ability to independently call for help.

An ECU can be set up for use while in bed, in the wheelchair, or both. There are one-room units available as well as multi-room units. Activation can be through the use of any type of a switch, through a sip and puff switch, or voice control.

There are advantages and disadvantages to all options. A thorough evaluation of your abilities and development of goals for use of the ECU are essential in order to select a unit that will meet your needs. Adequate training and technical support are also necessary to ensure successful use of the unit.

Funding for environmental control is often a challenge. Not all insurance companies or health-care providers pay for ECU. Your rehab team can help you brainstorm potential resources.

RESPIRATORY EQUIPMENT

Ventilators or continuous positive airway pressure (CPAP) may be required for some individuals with SCI. A suction machine or inexsufflator (coughalator) may be advised to assist with secretion removal and respiratory care. Your respiratory therapist, home health nurse, or medical equipment supplier will be able to answer questions about this equipment. A back up generator is essential for ventilator users. These are available at most hardware stores.

CONCLUSION

There is a tremendous amount of medical equipment advertised and available. Depending on your insurance or health-care provider, financial assistance may be available. It is important to consult your medical team to assist you in evaluating, recommending, and purchasing equipment to fit your specific needs. Remember, for all equipment, it is your responsibility to ensure safe operation and mechanical condition through regular maintenance.

People with spinal cord injuries face the same challenges to maintaining their health that their uninjured friends and neighbors do. Some areas of health that need your attention include vaccinations, colon cancer screening, male and female health issues, and satisfying sleep.

VACCINATIONS

It sometimes seems that the world is swarming with bacteria and viruses that are out to get us. For many of the common bacterial and viral infections, we have a great defense: vaccination.

Diphtheria/Tetanus

Everybody needs to stay current with diphtheria/tetanus vaccinations. The bacteria that causes tetanus (named *Clostridium tetani*) is everywhere in our environment. Our first line of defense against this bacteria is our skin. If our skin gets broken by a scrape, a cut, a puncture wound, or a tear, then this dangerous bacteria may get into our bodies and cause a severe disease, tetanus, that is often fatal.

Diphtheria is a disease that has virtually disappeared in the United States and Western Europe as the result of vaccination programs. In unvaccinated individuals, diphtheria occurs as a severe upper respiratory infection with extremely sore throat and can progress to closing the airway, severe cardiac infection, and death. The disease is starting to occur more frequently in Eastern Europe where vaccination programs have broken down in the last few years.

The best defense against these diseases is vaccination. After being immunized as children, adults should have a booster vaccination every 10 years. It's common in medical practice for people with traumatic injuries to be vaccinated if they haven't been vaccinated in the last 5 years.

Influenza

Influenza (flu) virus has built-in defenses that confound the effort to control it. The virus changes various characteristics on a frequent basis, so we need to be vaccinated every year against the flu. We tend to think of the flu as a trivial disease, but the worst epidemic in American history was the influenza epidemic of 1918. More people died in this epidemic than all of the combat deaths in that century combined.

People with respiratory diseases, elderly people, and people who work in health care are encouraged to get immunized every year. Since many people with spinal cord injury, especially quadriplegics, have respiratory impairments, you should be vaccinated every year.

There are also new drugs available to treat the flu if you get it, but they are most effective in the early stages of the illness. Therefore, if you get the flu, or think you might be getting the flu, it's best to call your doctor right away, so you can get the medicine you may need to prevent a severe case.

Pneumococcus

Pneumonia is the sixth leading cause of death in the United States. The most common cause of bacterial pneumonia is a bacteria named *Streptococcus Pneumoniae*. There are more than 90 strains of these bacteria, but vaccine is available to help prevent pneumonia from about 95 percent of them. Authorities recommend that people with chronic illnesses, especially respiratory diseases, and elderly people receive the vaccine. People with SCI, especially people with quadriplegia, often have respiratory impairments, so it is recommended that they receive this vaccine as well. People who receive the vaccine should have repeat vaccinations about every six years.

COLON CANCER SCREENING

Colon cancer is a common form of cancer in the United States. Fifteen percent of all cancer deaths are caused by colon cancer. The disease affects 2 out of every 1,000 people. There is no definitive way of preventing colon cancer. Factors that contribute to prevention are low fat, high fiber diet and regular bowel movements. Factors associated with an increased risk of colon cancer are colorectal polyps, cancer elsewhere in the body, a family history of colon cancer, ulcerative colitis, granulomatous colitis, and immune deficiency disorders.

If you have a family history of colon cancer, you should have your stool tested for hidden blood every year after you are 40 years old. If you don't have a family history, you should be checked every year after you are 50 years old. The test involves taking a small amount of stool and smearing it on a special card that you will be given (or receive in the mail) from your health-care providers. You return this card to them and they can then test to see if there is any blood present in your stool.

Factors that can cause this test to be less accurate include:

- Bleeding gums following a dental procedure
- Eating of red meat within 3 days
- Eating of fish, turnips, or horseradish

Drugs that can cause false positive results due to bleeding in the stomach and intestines include blood thinners, aspirin, colchicine, iron supplements in large doses, anti-inflammatory drugs, and corticosteroids. Other drugs that can cause false positive measurements include oxidizing drugs (such as iodine, bromides, and boric acid) and reserpine.

Large amounts of vitamin C can cause false negative results.

Bleeding hemorrhoids can cause false positive readings on this test and for people with SCI, if their bowel care is very vigorous or they are constipated and have hard stool, this may cause some minor bleeding in the rectum that can give a false positive reading.

To control for the possibility of false positive results, the test is normally repeated on three consecutive days.

If it is discovered that you have blood hidden in your stool, you should be referred to doctors who specialize in stomach and intestinal diseases (gastroenterologists) to have a colonoscopy or some other study performed. A colonoscopy is a test where a fiber optic tube is threaded up into your colon so the doctors can see the lining and identify any abnormalities by examination.

Colon cancer that is identified early is easily treatable with surgery and the chances of being cured of the disease are very good. If you are within the age guidelines given above (after you are 40 or 50) and your doctor does not offer you this test, ASK FOR IT!

GENDER-SPECIFIC HEALTH ISSUES

There are health issues that are specific to men and to women. People with SCI need to be aware of these problems and take the same steps that able-bodied people take to prevent them or at least to recognize them early.

Female Health Issues

Breast Cancer

It is estimated that one out of eight or nine women will develop breast cancer in the course of her life. The occurrence of breast cancer increases dramatically over the age of 30.

Some studies have indicated that diet may have an impact on the occurrence of the disease. Breast cancer appears to be more likely to develop in women whose diet is very high in fat. Older women who are overweight also seem to have a greater risk. Some scientists believe that a low-fat diet, eating well-balanced meals with plenty of fruits and vegetables, and maintaining ideal weight can lower the risk of breast cancer.

Other risk factors include having a family history of breast cancer, particularly in mother or sisters; a past medical history of breast cancer, ovarian cancer, uterine cancer, or colon cancer; early menarche (start of menstruation before age 12) or late menopause (after age 55); no pregnancies or a first pregnancy after age 30; and radiation exposure. Post-menopausal estrogen therapy and oral contraceptive use (such as estrogens and progestin oral contraceptives) were considered possible risk factors, but the majority of recent studies do not confirm such risk.

As with colon cancer and most other forms of cancer, the chances of successful treatment of breast cancer are best if the disease is detected early. The best practices for early detection include monthly breast self-exam after the age of 20 and yearly mammograms for women over 40.

Breast Self Exam (BSE)

Women should examine their breasts for lumps every month, at the same time after their period (menstruation). Just before menstruation and during pregnancy, a woman's breasts may be somewhat lumpy and more tender. If you are taking hormones, ask your doctor about when to perform BSE.

For women with SCI, there may be problems with sufficient hand function to complete this examination. Where this is the case, an attendant or family member should perform this examination for them. It would be important to have the same person performing this examination from month to month so that he or she may easily recognize any changes in the breast tissue.

To do BSE perform the following steps:

• Lie down; flatten your right breast by placing a pillow under your right shoulder. Place your right arm behind your back. You can also examine your breast when you are upright in the shower, using soap for lubrication.

• Use the fingertips (the most sensitive part of your hand for touch) of your middle three fingers. Feel for lumps using a circular, rubbing motion in small dime-sized circles without lifting your fingers. You can use powder, oil, or lotion to lubricate your hands to make this easier.

• Start with light pressure, move to medium pressure, and then use firm pressure to examine different levels of breast tissue.

• Completely examine all of the breast and chest area up under your armpit and up to the collarbone and all the way over to your shoulder.

- Use a pattern to insure that you examine the whole breast. This pattern could be parallel lines running from your shoulder toward your legs, concentric circles starting at the outside of your breast and moving inward toward the nipple, or you can use wedges, starting at the edges and moving toward the nipple in small wedge-shaped sections all around your breast. Whatever pattern you use, be sure to check the "tail" of the breast that runs up under your armpit.

- After you have completely examined your right breast, then examine your left breast using the same method.

- You should also examine your breasts in a mirror when you are upright looking for any changes in size or contour, dimpling of the skin, or spontaneous nipple discharge.

If you identify any changes in your breast tissue, in size or contour, any dimpling, or nipple discharge you need to be seen by your doctor soon.

Cervical Cancer

The third most common form of cancer in women is cervical cancer. Two to three percent of women over 40 will develop some form of cervical cancer. The cause of cervical cancer is unknown but factors that contribute to the development of cervical cancer include multiple sexual partners, early onset of sexual activity (less than 18 years), or early childbearing (less than 16 years). Sexually transmitted diseases, specifically Human papilloma virus (genital warts), HIV infection, and genital herpes, also appear to increase the risk of cervical cancer.

It is now known that women who were exposed to the drug DES (Diethylstilbestrol) in

utero are at risk for developing certain rare vaginal and cervical cancers along with many other abnormalities of the uterine, cervical, and vaginal tissues. DES is a drug that was once thought to prevent miscarriages. Unfortunately, the risks of taking DES were not known and between 1940 and the early 1970s, many pregnant women received the drug in hopes of preventing any suspected miscarriages. Clinical studies have shown the risk of cancer among the daughters born to women who were taking the drug to be around 4 in 1,000.

Cervical cancer may take years to develop. Initially, subtle changes develop in superficial cells of the cervix. Then the condition progresses to "dysplasia," which is the presence of pre-cancerous cells. These can then progress to superficial cancer (noninvasive) and then to invasive cancer that can spread to other abdominal organs.

Strategies to prevent cervical cancer include deferring sex until a person is 18 years old, monogamy, and safer sexual behaviors.

A routine pelvic examination, including a Pap smear, should be performed yearly beginning at the onset of sexual activity, or by the age of 20 in non-sexually active women. Pap smears detect abnormalities in the cells of the cervix, thus alerting the physician that further tests may need to be done. Early detection allows treatment to begin before cancer has actually developed.

Male Health Issues

Testicular Cancer

Cancer of the testicles accounts for only about 1 percent of all cancers in men. It is, however, the most common form of cancer in men between 18 and 25 years of age. Usually only one testicle is affected.

The cause of testicular cancer is not known but the known risk factors include:

- Uncorrected undescended testicles in infants and young boys
- A family history of testicular cancer
- Having an identical twin with testicular cancer
- Viral infections
- Injury to the scrotum

In the very early stages, testicular cancer may have no symptoms but when there are symptoms, they include:

- Small painless lump in testicle
- Enlarged testicle
- Feeling of heaviness in the testicle or groin
- Pain in the testicle
- A change in the way the testicle feels
- Enlarged male breasts and nipples
- Blood or fluid suddenly accumulating in the scrotum

Testicular cancer is almost always curable if it is found and treated early. The testicle is removed surgically. One testicle is sufficient for fully normal sexual functioning.

The American Academy of Family Physicians Subcommittee for Male Patients recommends learning testicular self-examination (TSE) between the ages of 13 and 18.

To perform TSE, examine each testicle gently with both hands. The index and middle fingers should be placed underneath the testicle while the thumbs are placed on top. Roll the testicle gently between the thumbs and fingers. It should feel smooth and have no bumps.

On the backside of the testicle you will feel a soft, ropy, tube-like structure. This is called the epididymis and should not be confused with a lump. Follow the epididymis up with your fingers until it enters the body. It should have the same consistency along its whole length.

If you have severe testicular pain, you should seek medical care urgently (this is more likely to be an infection or a physical problem rather than cancer, but it can be dangerous).

If there are any lumps, enlargements, swelling, or change in consistency or any sense of heaviness or pain, you should talk to your doctor. If there is an enlargement of the breasts and nipples or a sudden feeling of puffiness in the scrotum, you should also see a doctor.

You should practice TSE at least monthly or as directed by your doctor. Men with quadriplegia may need to have a family member or an attendant perform TSE for them. It is best if the same person performs the test from month to month in order to identify changes.

Prostate Health

We are hearing more and more about the dangers of prostate gland problems in men. Enlargement of the prostate gland, called benign prostatic hyperplasia (BPH), occurs in most men. Eighty percent of men over 40 and 95 percent of men over 80 have some degree of BPH. Eunuchs (men who have lost their testicles) do not develop BPH. This is the only know strategy for prevention of BPH and is, obviously, not recommended.

The biggest problems associated with BPH are changes in urination:

- Urgency (feeling a sudden strong urge to urinate)
- Frequency (having to urinate more often than normal)
- Urinary retention (not emptying the bladder completely)

In men with SCI, there can be increasing difficulty inserting a catheter and increased occurrence of bleeding and trauma from inserting a catheter. A special kind of catheter called a coudé tipped catheter often helps to go into the bladder through an enlarged prostate gland.

There are surgical procedures that can be done to help with prostate problems and there are medicines that you can take to help with this as well. Be sure to discuss this with your doctor if you suspect that you are having problems with an enlarged prostate gland.

Prostate cancer is a more serious problem. It is the third most common cause of death from cancer in all men and the most common cause of death from cancer in men over the age of 75. The incidence is greatest in African American men over 60 years old. Increased incidence is also associated with farmers, tire workers, painters, and men exposed to cadmium. The lowest incidence occurs in Japanese men and vegetarians.

The precise cause of prostate cancer and how to prevent it are not known. Adopting a vegetarian, low-fat diet or one that mimics the traditional Japanese diet may lower risk.

The key to survival is early detection. It is recommended by some healthcare organizations that men over 40 or 50 have a yearly rectal exam and a yearly laboratory test for the level of prostate specific antigen (PSA) in the blood stream. A normal level of PSA is 4 nanograms per milliliter. A PSA greater then 10 nanograms per milliliter requires further diagnostic testing. Values between 4 and 10 can be the result of BPH or prostatitis (an infection of the prostate gland).

Many men find rectal exams unpleasant and distasteful, but it is in their best interest to tough it out and have it done. Ninety-five percent of the changes in the prostate gland can be felt by the examiner during a rectal exam and this exam, coupled with PSA levels, can

identify prostate cancer at the earliest (and treatable) stages.

Breast Cancer

Both men and women can develop breast cancer. About 10 percent of cases of breast cancer each year occur in men. Consequently, men need to be aware of strategies for early detection as well as women.

AND A BEDTIME STORY

Satisfactory sleep time is an important element of a quality lifestyle. Human beings cycle through five different stages of sleep in the course of a typical night. There is the sleep pattern associated with dreaming, called rapid eye movement (REM) sleep because the eyes move through alternating cycles of slow and rapid movement during this stage. There are also four increasingly deepening sleep rhythms known as non-REM stage 1 through stage 4 sleep. In a normal night, the first half of the night is marked by long periods in deep non-REM sleep and the last half by long periods of REM sleep.

One interesting fact about sleep is that people's cycles tend to run in 25-hour cycles (not 24 hours to match a single day); that's why we sometimes feel the need to catch up on sleep on the weekends and why Mondays are so bleak for some people—because they have to get up much earlier than their internal clock would indicate.

Spinal cord injury may have subtle impacts on sleep patterns. Able-bodied people have a decrease in urine output during the hours of sleep, whereas people with SCI have a steady or even an increased level of urine output at night. This means that people who use intermittent catheterization for their bladder program need to be careful to reduce the amount of fluid they take in after dinner and may need to get up once during the night to catheterize themselves. One study that compared the time use patterns of men with SCI to able-bodied men found that men with SCI spent a little more time each day sleeping than the other people in the study.

Two factors that can cause difficulty sleeping are disrupted daily rhythms and aging. As we age, our sleep patterns change. We spend less time each night in deep non-REM sleep and we also have less REM sleep. Total sleep time may stay the same or even increase a little with aging, but our sense of feeling rested and refreshed after sleep diminishes with age. Also, changes in our daily rhythms—when we eat, when we try to sleep, and when we get up—can change our sense of rest and refreshment and even lead to difficulties falling or staying asleep.

Drugs aren't much help. Although some drugs may initially make falling asleep easier, they have a bad effect on the depth and quality of sleep. If they are used over a long period of time, they may make falling asleep even more difficult that it would have been otherwise. Many people try using alcoholic drinks to help with sleep, but although alcohol may initially make people feel sleepy, it has a very disruptive effect on the quality and quantity of sleep

So, in order to have the best quality of sleep, it's important to set and keep to a reasonably stable schedule. Get ready for bed at the same time at night. Develop and follow routines for getting ready for bed. Make sure that your bedroom can be darkened during your sleep periods. If there are problems with noises waking you, try using some form of "white noise" like table fans or recordings of wind and water sounds.

There are two medical conditions that can have an effect on your sleep. If you suspect that you have either of these, it's important to see your doctor. The first of these conditions is depression. With serious depression, people actually may sleep much more than eight hours a day, but they don't feel refreshed or energized after sleep. They may fall asleep easily enough at night but wake up in the early morning hours and have difficulty falling asleep again. If you experience sleep problems like this or a general absence of joy and pleasure in life, you should consult with your doctor. The drugs to treat depression have increased in quality and there is real hope of improved mood and improved sleep patterns.

Another disease that affects sleep is called sleep apnea. In sleep apnea, people actually stop breathing for brief periods when they are asleep at night. Their blood oxygen levels drop until they startle awake feeling anxious about insufficient air. These people most often snore loudly and their bed partners often are troubled by the uneven pattern of their breathing. People with sleep apnea are deprived of adequate rest and are often sleepy during the day. They fall into a doze readily during the day.

In the able-bodied population and probably among people with paraplegia, the risk factors for this condition are being male, getting older, and being overweight. Many people with quadriplegia have this condition without the normal risk factors. We don't really know why quads have this problem but a number of them do.

Risks associated with sleep apnea include high blood pressure, heart problems, and stroke. Another big problem is automobile accidents, since people with sleep apnea often fall asleep at the wheel. If you think you might have sleep apnea, there are some treatments that your doctor can use to try and help you. If you suspect you have this problem, exercise extreme caution when you are driving.

Glossary

This glossary of terms, lingo, and abbreviations is here for your use. It not only pertains to the contents of this manual, but also to the word usage you will hear during rehabilitation. You may wish to look these terms over to get a feel for SCI service terminology.

A

Abdominal binder
A cloth and elastic support worn wrapped around the abdomen to provide support for the abdominal wall muscles.

Acute stage
The time right after your injury when you are in the hospital and may have many kinds of medical problems.

Adaptive equipment
Equipment that is used to help adapt your environment to your personal needs. Examples include ramps, splints to hold pens or forks, and hand controls to drive vehicles.

ADL—activities of daily living
Self-care activities such as bathing, dressing, toileting, eating, grooming, etc.

Advocate
Someone who goes to bat for you and represents your best interests in a given situation.

Airways management
Methods to help you get the air you need into your lungs.

Anemia
A lack of red blood cells to carry oxygen to the tissues of the body.

Apartment
See Independent Living Unit.

Appliance
A device used to perform or help you perform a certain activity.

ASIA classification of spinal cord injury
The ASIA classification system uses standardized muscle testing and sensory examination to determine the level of spinal cord injury and predict the amount of preserved muscle function.

Assumption
Something that is taken to be right without proof or demonstration.

Atherosclerosis
Thickening of artery walls, hardening of the arteries.

Atrophy
A condition in which muscles diminish in size due to lack of stimulation from nerves.

Attendant
An individual (family, friend, paid staff, etc.) hired to assist with household tasks or personal care on a routine basis.

Automobile adaptive equipment
Items and/or devices necessary to permit the safe operation of or the ability to get in and out of an automobile or other types of vehicles.

B

Bedridden
Being confined to bed for medical treatment.

Bladder dysfunction
General term used to describe changes in the urinary bladder's ability to store and empty urine.

Bowel care
The procedure for starting and completing a bowel movement.

Bowel program
The total, individualized management plan to regularly empty the colon of stool. It includes diet, exercise, medication, and regularly scheduled bowel care.

Braces
Splints used to support, align, or hold parts of your body in correct position.

C

Capillary
A fine vessel that carries blood to tissues

Carbohydrates
Sugar and starches, a primary source of energy in the average U.S. diet. Complex carbohydrates (beans, peas, nuts, seeds, fruits, vegetables, whole grain breads, and cereals) supply fiber and many essential nutrients as well as calories.

Caregiver
General term used to describe any person who gives you physical, emotional, psychological, or social care.

Cath
Slang for catheterization.

Catheterization
Inserting a small special tube into your bladder to empty urine.

Cervical
Refers to conditions or things associated with the levels of your spine at the neck; also refers to the cervix, the necklike end of the uterus.

Cholesterol
A waxy-like, non-fat substance found in blood that is made by your liver or taken in from food sources of animal origin.

Chronic pain
Pain that has usually been present longer than six months and is out of proportion of physical and laboratory test results, for which pain medication does not work, and that becomes central to the lifestyle of the sufferer.

Chux
Absorbent pads used to protect a mattress, also known as "blue pads.

Cirrhosis
A disease of the liver aggravated by excessive alcohol consumption.

Clothing allowance
An annual sum of money specified by Congress to be paid to each veteran who, because if his or her service-connected disability, wears or uses a prosthetic or orthotic appliance (including a wheelchair) that tends to wear out or tear the clothing.

Contractures
Permanent limitation of joint movement usually due to not doing range of motion exercises, poor positioning, and/or severe spasms.

Contraindicated, contraindication
Bad for your health; a symptom, condition, or medication whose presence indicates some other treatment or medication should not be used.

Credé
A method of emptying the bladder by firm pressure on the abdomen with the hands to push the urine out.

D

Decubitus ulcer
Bed sore, pressure sore, pressure ulcer—a reddened area or open sore usually found on the skin over bony areas such as your hipbone or tailbone. Too much pressure on those areas usually causes them.

Digital stimulation
Gentle movement of a gloved finger in a circular pattern in the rectum to relax the sphincter muscle so that stool may pass during bowel care.

Discharge planning
See Chapter 21

Dosage
The amount of medication you should take and when to take it.

Drugs
Substances that cause effects on the body or mind. This includes both medications you take to get better and substances that are abused.

E

Edema
Fluid collecting in a given area of the body, causing swelling.

Eligibility
The determination of whether you qualify for certain entitlement programs. VA benefit payments are based on certain facts, including your period of service, whether you had an honorable or other discharge from the service, income guidelines, and a documented physical disability.

Embolus
A thrombus, or blood clot, that has broken loose and is passing freely through the bloodstream.

EMG—electromyogram
A test to find out how your nerves and muscles are working, using electronic equipment.

Evaluation
The careful study of something to determine its significance or value.

Extension
Unbending of a joint, for example, straightening your arm.

Extremity
A medical term referring to your arm or leg. Upper extremity includes your arm, forearm, and hand; lower extremity includes your thigh, lower leg, and foot.

F

Fabricate
To construct, assemble, or manufacture.

Flaccid
Lacking muscle tone.

Flexion
Bending of a joint, such as bending your leg at the knee.

Foley
Short for a foley catheter, a tube used to continuously drain urine from your bladder.

G

Gait
Description of an individual's style of walking.

H

Halo
A metal ring worn around your head used to treat broken necks. When used with a plastic vest, this keeps your neck and body straight.

HBHC—hospital based home care
The service offered by the hospital that tends to the care of people in their own homes.

Health promotion
Those activities and attitudes that help you live a healthy life.

Health risks
Those things, such as living conditions, heredity, attitudes, or activities, that increase your chances for poor health.

Hubbard tank
A tank of water used for exercise or treatment of pressure sores.

Hygiene
Condition or practices leading to health; usually used in reference to personal cleanliness.

Hypersensitive
Excessively sensitive, a condition in which there is exaggerated response by the body to stimulation such as touching, stretching, or movement.

I

ICP
See intermittent catheterization program

Impaction
Something that gets lodged in and clogs a space, such as an impaction of the bowel.

Incentive spirometer
A device used to build up lung volume and control.

Incontinence
Inability to exercise voluntary control over your bowel or bladder, leading to leaking or other accidents.

Independent Living Unit
A full apartment on the SCI unit where patients can test new skills and be evaluated on what they have learned in therapy sessions.

Intermittent catheterization program
ICP or cath—a routine program by which the bladder is emptied at regular intervals by catheterization to prevent urinary accidents and infections.

Involuntary
Independent of the will; not under voluntary control.

L

Ligament
A band or sheet of fibrous tissue connecting two or more bones, cartilages, or other structures.

LPN—licensed practical nurse
A person trained and licensed to provide routine nursing care.

Lumbar
Refers to a condition or thing in the area of the mid to lower back.

Lung capacity
The volume of air you can breathe and your lungs can hold.

M

MD—doctor of medicine
Someone who has completed four years of medical school. May be an intern, resident, or staff doctor.

Medical history
The important information about your (and your family's) past and present health.

Medication—medicine
A therapeutic substance you take that is prescribed by your doctor or purchased "over the counter."

N

NA—nursing assistant
Someone who assists nurses by performing routine, nonclinical tasks, such as serving meals and making beds.

Neurogenic
Refers to a condition or thing that is controlled by nerves or in which the control by the nerves has been damaged.

Nutrition
The food you eat and how your body uses it to live, grow, keep healthy, and get the energy you need for work and recreation.

O

Occupational therapy or therapist—OT
The profession or professional that focuses on the range of motion; strength; and coordination of fine, or small, movement of muscles and joints, with or without adaptive devices. The end result is to enable you to perform ADL tasks or various vocational skills.

Oral
Pertaining to or taken through your mouth.

Orthosis, orthotics
A device applied to the exterior of the body to support, aid, and align the body and limbs or to influence motion by assisting, resisting, blocking, or unloading part of the body weight. These devices may include, but are not limited to, braces, binders, corsets, belts, and trusses.

Orthostatic hypotension
A form of low blood pressure that occurs in a standing posture.

P

Pandemic
An epidemic that affects an unusually large area and population.

Para—paraplegia
Paralysis of the legs and lower body.

Paralysis
The inability to control movement of a part of your body.

Paraparesis
Incomplete paralysis or weakness of the legs only.

Personality
Thoughts, feelings, and behaviors that are specific to an individual, often representing a particular pattern or style of life.

Physiotherapy, physical therapy, therapist—PT
The profession or professional that deals with the strength, coordination, and range of motion of gross movements of your muscles and joints.

Pneumonia
Inflammation of the lung tissue characterized by filling of air sacks with fluids. Most cases are due to infection by bacteria or viruses.

Pressure reliefs
Changes in position in the wheelchair or bed to let your skin rest and increase circulation of blood flow in the buttocks or areas of pressure; used to prevent decubitus ulcers.

Primary care
The medical care of routine illnesses such as colds, flu, etc.

Prone
Lying flat on your stomach.

Prosthesis
An artificial substitute for a missing body part.

Prosthetic appliances
All aids, appliances, parts, or accessories that are required to replace, support, or substitute for a deformed, weakened, or missing anatomical portion of the body. Artificial limbs, terminal devices, stump socks, braces, hearing aids and batteries, cosmetic facial or body restorations, eyeglasses, mechanical or motorized wheelchairs, orthopedic shoes, and similar items are included under this broad term.

Psychological
Related to mental and emotional factors that influence behavior (motivation, awareness, personality, etc.).

PT—physical therapy, physical therapist
See Physiotherapy.

Pulmonary
Having to do with your lungs and breathing.

Q

Quad—quadriplegia, tetraplegia
Paralysis of all four limbs.

Quadriparesis
Weakness or incomplete paralysis involving the arms and legs.

R

Range of motion—ROM
An arc of movement of a joint of your body, also used to refer to the exercises done to maintain and increase the arc of movement.

Registered nurse—RN
A professional, trained and authorized by a state board of nursing examiners, who plans and provides nursing care. Your primary care planner is usually an RN.

Rehab—rehabilitation
The process of doing away with, adapting to, or compensating for disabilities.

Residual
In the case of bladder voiding, urine left in the bladder after voiding has taken place.

Respiratory
Having to do with breathing.

Respiratory therapy, therapist—RT
The profession or professional that centers on therapy of the lungs and breathing.

S

Sacral
Refers to a condition or thing in the area at the lowest part of your spine around your tailbone.

SCI—spinal cord injury
An injury to the back or neck causing damage to the spinal cord, leading to paralysis.

Sensation
Physical feelings of vibration, touch, pain, hot and cold, or awareness of where a body part is in space.

Side effects
The effects of something, usually medication, that are different from the reason for which it was originally planned.

Smoker's robot
A mechanical device that holds a cigarette safely away from the smoker. The cigarette can then be smoked through a piece of tubing. "Safely" refers to prevention of burns from falling ashes and embers, not the toxic effects of cigarette smoking.

Spasm
A sudden, often uncontrolled, contraction of a muscle; a muscle jerk.

Spasticity
Movement in your arms and legs due to muscle spasms that may occur as a result of spinal cord injury. It may be somewhat controllable. Spasticity may also be useful in maintaining muscle size, bone strength, and circulation.

Spine immobilizers
Braces or devices that keep you from moving your back or neck.

Spine stabilization
Use of a brace or device that aids in supporting or stabilizing your back or neck.

Splint

A rigid or flexible appliance used for the fixation (holding in place) or support of a displaced or movable part of the body.

Stones

Solid, hard masses that can become stuck in the urinary track and block normal urine drainage from the kidney or bladder.

Suctioning

Removal of mucous from the throat and lungs by a small tube attached to suction.

Support system

The people who are important to you because they strengthen your emotional, physical, and social well-being. They include your family, friends, co-workers, neighbors, members of your church, or veterans group.

T

Tenodesis

The action of fingers and thumb pinching together when wrist is bent upwards.

Tetraplegia

See quadriplegia.

Therapy

Treatment of diseases, disorders, or disabilities.

Thoracic

Refers to a condition or thing in the region of the spine at the chest or mid-back level.

Thrombus

A blood clot anchored somewhere in the bloodstream.

TRS—therapeutic recreation specialist

The person responsible for your recreational therapy.

U

Urinalysis

A sampling test of urine to evaluate the contents of the urine and check for problems.

Urinary system

The body parts that turn wastes into urine, store it, and get rid of it. Kidneys filter blood to wash it clean and make the urine. Ureters are tubes to bring the urine from the kidneys to the bladder. The bladder is a dynamic storage tank for the urine. The urethra is a tube to bring the urine from the bladder to the outside.

V

VA—U.S. Department of Veterans Affairs

The branch of the federal government responsible for providing health care and other benefits to eligible veterans of the armed forces.

VBA—Veterans Benefits Administration

Branch of the U.S. Department of Veterans Affairs responsible for administering compensation and pension benefits to eligible veterans.

Ventilator

A piece of equipment that helps you to breathe when you cannot do it yourself.

Vocational

Work or job-related activities.

Voc rehab—vocational rehabilitation

Developing skills to improve work habits or to increase employment potential.

Void

To empty the bladder.

VRS—vocational rehabilitation specialist

The person who assists you in developing skills and determining changes or improvements in your job or vocational status.

Resource Organizations

The following organizations address a wide range of goals, objectives, programs, services, and interests concerned with spinal cord injury.

Christopher Reeve Paralysis Foundation
500 Morris Avenue
Springfield, NJ 07081
(800) 225-0292
www.apacure.org

A merger of the American Paralysis Association and the Christopher Reeve Foundation. This foundation supports research to develop effective treatments and a cure for paralysis.

Association of Programs for Rural Independent Living
5903 Powdermill Road
Kent, OH 44240
(330) 678-7648
(330) 678-8467 TTY
(330) 678-7658 fax
www.april-rural.org

The Canadian Paraplegic Association (CPA)
1101 Prince of Wales Dr. Suite 230
Ottawa, Ontario K2C 3W7
(800) 720-4933
email: info@canparaplegic.org
www.canparaplegic.org

The CPA is concerned with every phase of rehabilitation of the spinal cord injured from initial trauma to lifelong adjustment.

Canine Companions for Independence (CCI)
P.O. Box 446
Santa Rosa, CA 95402-0446
(800) 572-2275
www.caninecompanions.org

CCI is a nonprofit organization that provides highly trained assistance dogs to people with disabilities and to professional caregivers.

Disabled American Veterans (DAV)
P.O. Box 14301
Cincinnati, OH 45250-0301
(859) 441-7300
www.dav.org

This veterans service organization provides assistance to all veterans and members of their families. Membership is open to all disabled veterans.

Easter Seals
230 W. Monroe St., Suite 1800
Chicago, IL 60606
(800) 221-6827; (312) 726-6200
(312) 726-4258 TTY
www.easter-seals.org

A national organization with local chapters. Serves all people with disabilities, comprehensive and individualized to meet each client's needs.

Helping Hands

541 Cambridge Street

Boston, MA 02134

(617) 787-4419

www.helpinghandsmonkeys.org

Helping Hands is a nonprofit organization dedicated to improving life for quadriplegic individuals by training capuchin monkeys to assist them with daily activities.

The Job Accommodation Network (JAN)

West Virginia University

P.O. Box 6080

Morgantown, WV 26506-6080

(800) 526-7234

www.janweb.icdi.wvu.edu.

JAN is not a job placement service, but an international toll-free consulting service that provides information about job accommodations and the employment of people with disabilities.

National Council on Independent Living

1916 Wilson Boulevard, Suite 209

Arlington, VA 22201

(703) 525-3406

(703) 525-4153 TTY

(703) 525-3409 fax

www.ncil.org

NCIL is a membership organization that advances the independent living philosophy and advocates for the human rights of and services for people with disabilities.

The National Institute on Disability and Rehabilitation Research

400 Maryland Ave, SW

Washington, DC 20202-2572

(202) 205-8134

(202) 205-4475 TTY

www.ed.gov/about/offices/list/osers/nidrr/index.html

This federal agency supports the model regional SCI care system and related research efforts. It administers grant programs including the Rehabilitation Research and Training Centers.

National Institute of Neurological Disorders and Stroke (NINDS)

NIH Neurological Institute

P.O. Box 5801

Bethesda, MD 20824

(800) 352-9424; (301) 496-5751

(301) 468-5981 TTY

www.ninds.nih.gov

Part of the National Institutes of Health, NINDS conducts, fosters, coordinates, and guides research on the causes, prevention, diagnosis, and treatment of neurological disorders and stroke.

National Organization on Disability

910 Sixteenth Street, NW, Suite 600

Washington, DC 20006

(202) 293-5960

(202) 293-5968 TTY

www.nod.org

The National Organization on Disability promotes full and equal participation of America's 54 million men, women, and children with disabilities in all aspects of life.

National Spinal Cord Injury Association (NSCIA)
6701 Democracy Blvd., Suite 300-9
Bethesda, MD 20817
(800) 962-9629
www.spinalcord.org

This organization provides advocacy, peer support, and other services to individuals with SCI, their families, and health-care providers. It supports research aimed at improving care for people with SCI and developing a cure. The Foundation has chapters in many states. Each chapter can help provide information about local resources, social activities, and advocacy.

Paralyzed Veterans of America
801 Eighteenth Street, NW
Washington, DC 20006
(202) 872-1300
www.pva.org

The Paralyzed Veterans of America, a congressionally chartered veterans service organization, works to improve the quality of life for individuals with an SCI through research, education, and advocacy for health care, civil rights, and opportunities of its members and all Americans with a spinal cord dysfunction.

Office of Disability Employment Policy (ODEP)
U.S. Department of Labor
200 Constitution Avenue, NW, Room S-1303
Washington, DC 20210
(202) 693-7880
(202) 693-7881 TTY
www.dol.gov/odep

This committee communicates, coordinates, and promotes public and private efforts to enhance the employment of people with disabilities.

Spinal Cord Injury Information Network
University of Alabama at Birmingham
Department of Physical Medicine and Rehabilitation
619 19th Street South SRC529
Birmingham, AL 35249-7330
(205) 934-3334
TTY: (205) 934-4642
www.spinalcord.uab.edu

UAB hosts a model spinal cord injury center, supporting research and patient education projects. The Rehabilitation Research and Training Center conducts research and training in the prevention and treatment of secondary conditions of spinal cord injury. Under a grant from the National Institute on Disability and Rehabilitation Research, they maintain a website that provides links to educational and research information.

University of Washington Department of Rehabilitation Medicine
Box 356490
Seattle, WA 98195-6490
(206) 543-3600
depts.washington.edu/rehab/

The website of the University of Washington School of Medicine's Department of Rehabilitation Medicine offers extensive resources for researchers, health-care providers, and consumers.